GOD-GIVEN REMEDIES FOR EVERYDAY AILMENTS

1,001 Amazing Secrets for Seniors That Prevent and Reverse Disease — Naturally

Publisher's Note

This book is intended for general information only. It does not constitute medical, legal, or financial advice or practice. The editors of FC&A have taken careful measures to ensure the accuracy and usefulness of the information in this book. While every attempt has been made to assure accuracy, errors may occur. Some websites, addresses, and telephone numbers may have changed since printing. We cannot guarantee the safety or effectiveness of any advice or treatments mentioned. Readers are urged to consult with their professional financial advisors, lawyers, and health care professionals before making any changes.

Any health information in this book is for information only and is not intended to be a medical guide for self-treatment. It does not constitute medical advice and should not be construed as such or used in place of your doctor's medical advice. Readers are urged to consult with their health care professionals before undertaking therapies suggested by the information in this book, keeping in mind that errors in the text may occur as in all publications and that new findings may supersede older information.

The publisher and editors disclaim all liability (including any injuries, damages, or losses) resulting from the use of the information in this book.

And He said to her, "Daughter, your faith has saved you;
go in peace and be healed of your affliction."
Mark 5:34

Table of Contents

Diabetes 105

Diarrhea 123

Dry skin 131

High cholesterol 231

Allergies

Sneezy, wheezy, itchy, and dopey — sounds like a line in a story-book. But this is certainly no fairy tale. These are the telltale signs of allergic rhinitis, a miserable reaction your body has to something in your environment, and a condition that affects about 60 million Americans. Whether seasonal or year-round, the symptoms can wreak havoc on your body as well as your social life. And although allergic rhinitis is commonly called hay fever, don't be fooled. There's rarely any hay or fever involved.

While you may have heard of allergic reactions to food, animal dander, bug stings, or medications, in the case of allergic rhinitis, the most common culprits are mold spores, dust, grasses, trees, and weeds. But all allergies, from peanuts to pollen, basically work the same way.

Step 1. You come in contact with an allergen, and your body mistakenly treats it as an invader.

Step 2. Your immune system produces antibodies that, in turn, cause your cells to release irritating chemicals like histamine to fight off this invader.

Step 3. The histamines and other substances cause inflammation and lead to a variety show of symptoms. Here's where you start to feel miserable. In the case of allergic rhinitis, you might experience a stuffy nose, itchy eyes, sneezing, a cough — the whole shebang.

Though scientists are discovering cutting-edge ways to put a lid on allergic inflammation, there is still no golden cure. For you, that means fighting back with the basics, specifically a healthy lifestyle. Here are a few interesting and practical tips to nip allergies in the bud — without ever leaving home.

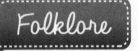

Allerlore —
don't fall for this 'remedy'

Some say Himalayan salt rocks produce negative ions that attract mold, dust, and pollen, cleaning the air in style. And that's how sellers of salt lamps are promoting their wares. But as far as seasonal allergies are concerned, scientists say no one has proven these salt lamps have any health benefits. If you want to set one up for decoration, go for it, but don't expect the lamp to zap your allergies.

6 ways to survive the sneezing season

Pollen-proof your wardrobe. Did you know wearing that moisture-wicking performance T-shirt on your afternoon walk can make your allergies worse? Synthetic fabrics rub together, creating a small electrical charge that attracts pollen.

According to experts, you should stick to cotton when you're out and about. This natural fiber can't hold an electric charge, so you won't gather more pollen as you go about your day.

Clear out allergens with a quick rinse. Take a shower at night and you'll wash the day's pollen from your skin, hair, and even your eyelashes. But have you paid attention to your nose lately?

Pollen and other allergens stick around by sticking to the mucus in your nasal passageways. Experts say try washing your nose in the shower. Just lean forward, rinse, and blow. Genius.

You can also use saline products, nasal bulbs, or Neti pots to flush out the bad stuff. If you want to make your own saline solution, the American Academy of Allergy, Asthma & Immunology (AAAAI) recommends mixing 3 teaspoons of iodide-free salt with 1 teaspoon of baking soda. When you're ready, add 1 teaspoon of the mixture to 1 cup of lukewarm distilled or boiled water.

Make a clean sweep of household triggers. Allergens may be running rampant in your home right now, but you'll never see them. Take dust mites, for instance. They are one of the biggest culprits, but measure a measly 1/4 millimeter. To put that in perspective, a credit card is about 1 millimeter thick. Pet dander and dust particles are microscopic, as well.

While you may not be able to see these irritants to get rid of them entirely, you can take steps to limit the amount in your home.

▸ Remove carpet if you can. It's a breeding ground for dust, pet dander, and the pollen you track in throughout the day.

▸ If you can't leave your pets outside, at least keep them out of bedrooms.

▸ Crank up the dehumidifier. Dust mites and mold love humidity.

▶ Use dust-proof mattress and pillow covers, and wash bed linens frequently in hot water.

Take the edge off allergies from the inside out. Probiotics are legendary for reviving gut health, but what does that have to do with the sniffles? Your tummy and intestines affect many parts of your body — even your allergy response.

Researchers looked at 23 studies examining the use of good bacteria for allergic rhinitis. They discovered a majority of those who took supplements or ate foods containing probiotics saw benefits, particularly improved symptoms or boosts in quality of life. Still, researchers want to see more studies before making recommendations. They have yet to pin down the best probiotic strains and doses for the job.

Probiotics probably won't replace standard allergy treatments, but if you want to give them a try, you'll also reap benefits for your digestion. Certain foods, such as miso soup, sauerkraut, pickles, dark chocolate, and yogurt with live active cultures, are natural sources of probiotics.

Soothe nose troubles with a zesty spice. Ah, the allergic salute — a quick swipe of the hand to relieve nose itch and stuffiness. Not all that socially acceptable. And really, wouldn't it be better if you could calm the sneezing and sniffling before it comes to this? New research published in *The Journal of Nutritional Biochemistry* says you can.

All it takes is a sprinkle of powdered ginger to slow down the production of antibodies that release histamines — the source of many allergy woes. At least it works on animals.

The good news is the study used small amounts of the same kind of powdered ginger you'll find in your kitchen. Unfortunately, scientists don't yet have an exact dosage for people. However, other studies that examined the effects of ginger on digestive symptoms, such as nausea, used up to 50 grams of the spice, or just under 2 ounces, with success.

So add a delightfully zingy taste to meat, seafood, vegetables, noodles, and rice. And while ginger is helping your nose, it's also opening your airways. Breathe easier knowing this spice is hard at work beating back inflammation and clearing up nasal troubles.

Get the buzz on local honey. Old wives' tale or proven home remedy? When it comes to honey for allergies, the answer may lie somewhere in between.

The theory is when you eat raw, local honey, you get small doses of pollen, which can help you build up a tolerance to seasonal allergies. The idea makes sense — after all allergy shots work the same way to desensitize your immune system. But here's what the critics have to say. The pollen that bees collect is not the kind that aggravates your allergies. That comes from grass, trees, and weeds, which are not pollinated by bees. And while tiny amounts of allergy-causing pollen may end up in raw honey by accident, it's not enough to do the job.

It's true, there's not much research to back up the claims — although lots of people say honey has brought them allergy relief. But here is what a small study out of Malaysia recently found. When allergy sufferers ate local, unprocessed honey in addition to taking an antihistamine, they had fewer symptoms — stuffy, itchy, runny nose and sneezing — compared to those taking the antihistamine alone. The researchers say honey may help control how hypersensitive you are to irritants on a cellular level.

Be aware that raw honey may cause allergic reactions in some people, so if you experience any unusual symptoms, stop taking it.

Outsmart food allergies with fiber

Who Knew?

An Australian study reports a high-fiber diet, along with the right amount of vitamin A, could help protect against food allergies by actually changing the type and amount of bacteria in your gut. Children, especially, are prone to food allergies, and the researchers believe if their diet falls short of these important nutrients, they could be at risk. No matter what your age, a healthy amount of fiber is good for your digestion and your immune system. So make sure you get enough by loading your plate with plenty of fruits and vegetables.

Food reactions often triggered by pollen woes

Do you get an itchy, tingly mouth when you nibble on carrots? What about a scratchy throat or swollen lips when you snack on peaches? You think you're allergic to raw fruits and veggies, but you may actually be experiencing oral allergy syndrome because you are allergic to birch pollen.

This condition, also called pollen-food syndrome, occurs when your immune system reacts to a food protein that is similar to a pollen you are allergic to. The good news is you may be able to eat the same fruits or vegetables in cooked form. That's because the proteins are changed by the heat, and your immune system isn't stirred up.

Symptoms are usually limited to your mouth and throat, and pass quickly, but if they make you uncomfortable, you can avoid problem foods. Here are some common allergens and their food triggers.

▸ Birch pollen: apples, almonds, carrots, celery, cherries, hazelnuts, kiwi, peaches, pears, plums

▸ Grass pollen: celery, melons, oranges, peaches, tomatoes

▸ Ragweed pollen: bananas, cucumbers, melons, sunflower seeds, zucchini

Buyer beware: 'hypoallergenic' may be all hype

Like many allergy sufferers, Darlene has a difficult time finding products that don't irritate her skin and cause other reactions. It doesn't help that items claiming to be hypoallergenic or fragrance-free still aggravate her symptoms. What gives? It turns out, those labels don't always mean what you expect. From makeup to bedding to puppies, hypoallergenic may be just another empty word.

The term "hypoallergenic" belongs entirely to the marketing world. The claim is not regulated by the Food and Drug Administration (FDA), which means companies can stick a hypoallergenic label on anything.

To find out how the claims stack up in run-of-the-mill goods, scientists put it to the test. They evaluated allergens in 187 products marketed as "hypoallergenic," "dermatologist recommended/tested," "fragrance free," or "paraben free." They found that 89 percent contained at least one allergen — the most common were preservatives and fragrances.

Nasal filters bring fast relief

New!

Want to keep allergens out of your nose? Put up a barrier. Maybe something less conspicuous than that surgical face mask. Why not coat each nostril with a beeswax-based balm designed to trap pollen before it reaches your nasal passages? Or puff a bit of natural cellulose powder into your nose, where it turns into a gel and absorbs allergens as they pass. These products have been around a while, and show some success. But you do have to reapply them frequently.

Now you can buy small disposable filters that sit inside your nostrils and screen allergens like grass pollen. According to studies, these nose masks reduce runny nose, itching, sneezing, throat irritation, and even watery eyes. Just be sure you put them in place before you're exposed to irritants.

Anxiety

"Anxiety does not empty tomorrow of its sorrow, but only empties today of its strengths," preached Charles Spurgeon in the 19th century. Nearly 200 years later, this philosophy is still relevant, since 75 percent of Americans feel some symptom of stress. Yet one out of five say they never do anything to relieve or manage it. Stressing about tomorrow is a habit that's hard to shake.

Calm your nerves to reverse aging. So what's the problem? A little anxiety won't kill you, right? Well, not so fast. Research links worrying to poor decision-making, chronic pain, and disease — like heart disease, dementia, and diabetes. And in fact, anxiety could shorten your life by three to five years. Here's how.

When researchers analyzed more than 2,300 people, they discovered those with anxiety disorders had shorter telomere length. Like the plastic tips on your shoelaces, telomeres are the DNA that cap the ends of your chromosomes, protecting them from unraveling. Telomeres naturally shorten as you age, eventually becoming so short your cells can no longer reproduce. This causes your tissues to deteriorate and die. That's why experts consider short telomeres a sign of cellular aging.

The telomeres in the anxious group equaled about three to five years of accelerated cell aging, compared to those without anxiety disorders. Surprisingly, those in the study who had learned to control their anxiety for at least 10 years, didn't have short telomeres. This suggests you could reverse the cellular aging process brought on by stress.

Need more incentive to get your anxiety under control? If you learn to respond to stress positively, you could lower the amount of inflammation in your body, and that's a major influence on long-term health.

Spot the source of your tension. First of all, it's important to identify where your uneasiness is coming from. Are you having trouble sleeping the night before a big presentation? Does your headache stem from upcoming bills? Is your blood pressure through the roof on account of lunch with your mother-in-law? Really examine your stress triggers and take steps to improve these situations.

Then take back today with any one of these simple and natural ways to calm your nerves.

9 tips to tame the anxiety beast

The edible fix for your jitters. Your gut has a long job description, and "second brain" is just one of its many titles. The millions of neurons in your stomach and intestines send signals straight to your noggin — signals that not only make you feel full, but also moody or satisfied. That's why researchers think probiotics — the "good" bacteria in your gut — may help anxiety and depression.

Among other things, probiotics raise your body's level of GABA (gamma-aminobutyric acid), a chemical messenger that helps control fear and anxiety. It's the same neurotransmitter that is mimicked in many anti-anxiety drugs. But unlike drugs, probiotics naturally encourage your body to make more GABA.

A recent study out of the College of William and Mary found that fermented foods, which are high in probiotics, helped people with social anxiety disorder control their symptoms. These foods include yogurt, kefir, miso soup, sauerkraut, pickles, and kimchi.

Your go-to tunes beat back tension. If you think your favorite melodies help calm you down, it's not just in your head. Researchers have actually put it to the test, and the results will be music to your ears.

Studies show music relieves depression, cuts down pain, and reduces anxiety during surgeries and dental treatments. Experts say your favorite tunes touch the emotional center of your brain, relaxing your mind and distracting you from your worries. Listening to those mellow jazz tunes you love may be just what you need when your mind starts spinning or your heart starts pounding.

You may get the same mood-boosting benefits by singing or going to a concert. The best part is you'll be singing a different tune with no pills, no side effects, and no worries.

The laughing cure — chuckle your stress away. "Laughter is an instant vacation," said comedian Milton Berle. And he's not the only one who thinks so.

What's so funny? The fact that laughter can dissolve stress, anxiety, and depression — even if it's forced. Experts say pretend cackling unleashes the same anti-stress hormones you release when you laugh for real. In one study, breast cancer patients participated in an hour-long program, where different activities encouraged loud, lengthy bouts of laughter. After just one session, they felt less anxious and depressed.

Now you can find laughter therapy clubs and even laughter-based exercise programs, which combine the beauty of laughter with the long-established mood benefits of exercise. For a quick pick-me-up, get together with a few of your funniest friends.

Tap into the healing power of pets. No question, a playful pooch can be a joy and a comfort, especially if you're feeling down or anxious. Experts say just turn to that little tail-wagger for some "bone"-a fide therapy.

Studies show interacting with a pet, particularly dogs, means less anxiety, depression, loneliness, and boredom. In addition, spending time with your beloved animals may lower your heart rate and blood pressure.

> Even if you don't own a pet, happy time can be just around the corner. Visit an animal shelter or volunteer to walk your neighbor's dog.

Being kind eases your mind. If you've ever felt anxious in a crowd, this one's for you. Simply helping people out on a regular basis can make you more comfortable whenever you interact with others.

In a recent study, researchers gathered together college students who suffered from social anxiety — those who felt shy, embarrassed, or uncomfortable meeting and interacting with others. For four weeks, one group regularly performed small, random acts of kindness, like doing the dishes for their roommate, mowing the neighbor's lawn, or donating to a charity. One group socialized while practicing deep breathing, and the final group simply wrote down events from their day.

The group that reached out to others ended up feeling less anxious in social situations and were also less likely to avoid them.

Try it yourself. If you get stressed when you go out, find little chores or tasks to do that benefits others or makes them happy. You'll reap the rewards, too.

Boost your mood with a little creativity. Adult coloring books are the new craze in America. Fans of this hobby claim it relieves stress and helps them relax. But is there any science behind getting crafty to fight anxiety?

While most evidence comes from personal testimonies, a few small studies do show that crafts such as knitting help calm anxiety. Many find that the repetitive motion and focus required for these tasks are quite soothing.

Doing crafts can take your mind off worries, quiet your nerves, and give you a sense of pride. So make time for what makes you happy, whether it's knitting, painting, or scrapbooking.

Take a moment to breathe. There's one remedy that can quell anxiety no matter where life takes you. And you're doing it right now — breathing.

Of course to get the most benefit, you may have to tweak your technique, to something called deep breathing, or abdominal breathing. It's a simple practice that increases oxygen to your brain and helps you calm down. Your heart beats slower, your muscles relax, and your blood pressure goes down.

It's so easy you can do it at your work desk or on your sofa at home. Count to five as you breathe in slowly through your nose. Make sure it's a nice deep breath that expands your chest and lower belly. Then, breathe out slowly through your mouth or nose. Try this at least 10 to 20 minutes each day.

Let nature relax, refresh, and restore. Ready for a stroll? Head for the park, not downtown. Take the green path, not the sidewalk.

Maybe soaking up the atmosphere of nature, which the Japanese call forest bathing, has always made you feel better, but now science proves it can lessen anxiety and negative thinking. A peaceful stroll through the woods may also lower symptoms of stress by balancing your heart rate, blood pressure, and stress hormones.

A walk in the woods can also be a spiritual experience. Take that time to engage in some private prayer, and it may restore your health if you're struggling with depression or anxiety.

Journal your way to joy. You can cut through stress and boost your mood in just 20 minutes a week. How? Simply start a gratitude journal, and write about positive aspects of your life. It will literally change your brain.

Researchers out of Indiana University found expressing thankfulness this way boosted activity in areas of the brain that deal with emotions — including loss, fear, and stress. People who did this for three weeks experienced less negativity and sparked even more feelings of gratitude. Plus, they continued to see results three months later.

Anti-anxiety herbs soothe stress naturally

The source of your anxiety may be hard to pinpoint, but its symptoms are easy to recognize. Spikes in your blood pressure, sleeplessness, and uncontrollable butterflies tell you your body is under stress. Interested in a natural solution?

Studies show your nose may be the key to relieving anxiety. And marjoram has received special attention. When researchers reviewed the records of more than 10,000 hospital patients, they found the scent of marjoram scored high marks for controlling anxiety and pain.

Experts say marjoram relaxes your nervous system and restores good blood pressure by dilating your arteries and small blood vessels. It's also a crowd favorite among those with sleep troubles caused by stress. This kitchen herb can truly do it all.

Need more reasons to love natural remedies? Here are four other herbs known for calming and soothing.

Lavender. It's one of the best-known herbs for relaxation, often drunk as a tea or used in massage. Add a few drops of lavender essential oil to your warm bath water to calm down and relieve stress.

Chamomile. This herb makes for classic bedtime tea. Studies show chamomile might help anxiety and insomnia as well as stomach upsets caused by stress.

Lemon balm. Comforting lemon balm tea tastes just as zesty and delicious as it sounds. It's often used to treat anxiety, depression, and stomach nerves.

Passionflower. Studies show passionflower relieves anxiety by increasing brain levels of a chemical called GABA (gamma-aminobutyric acid). Passionflower is often easier to find in combination with other herb products.

Talk to your doctor before using these herbs for extended periods of time, and be sure to check for interactions with any drugs you may already be taking.

Warning

Kava: the Pacific potion to avoid

Kava bars are cropping up across the U.S. But beware, this ancient Polynesian beverage has a murky safety history.

The root of the kava plant has been used in ceremonial drinks in the Pacific Islands for hundreds of years, yet it fell out of medical favor not long after studies showed evidence of dangerous side effects such as liver damage.

Supporters of trendy kava cafes say the drink relieves anxiety and helps you relax. While a number of studies agree, experts still warn against the dangers and say it's impossible to know what dose of kava might be safe.

Athlete's foot

Bob was thrilled to retire, but not long after, he noticed the skin on his feet was peeling, and he couldn't get rid of a maddening itch between his toes. Soon, it even hurt to walk.

No, he wasn't allergic to retirement. But his doctor told him about a surprising link. When Bob retired, he went back to an old hobby of his — swimming laps at the local pool. That's probably where he picked up athlete's foot, the cause of his painful skin problems.

Athlete's foot is a public affair. It's every gym-goer's worst nightmare, but you don't have to be sporty to get athlete's foot. It gets its name because the fungus that causes it loves warm and wet environments — like the sweaty feet of the average jock. That means public places like locker rooms, showers, and swimming pools are free game. And as Bob found out, going barefoot makes you vulnerable.

The fungus spreads easily through contact, but it doesn't have to be skin to skin. You can pass it along by sharing socks, sneakers, towels, even bed sheets.

Stubborn symptoms are tough to control. In addition to Bob's symptoms, your feet may develop blisters or a scaly red rash that stings or burns. Raw, moist skin between the toes is common, but the fungus can easily spread to the soles of your feet and your toenails. Not to mention, make them smell.

Unfortunately, this stubborn fungus usually doesn't go away on its own. And once the infection reaches your nails, it's even harder to get rid of. Over-the-counter creams and natural remedies will usually get the job done. Just make sure you continue the treatment for one or two weeks after symptoms disappear. Fungus likes to linger.

Simple ways to sidestep the fungus. These days, Bob is more mindful of his foot health. He gives his friends this advice about easy ways to avoid athlete's foot.

▸ Put on shoes in public places. Even if you feel silly wearing shoes in the shower, flip flops are better than fungus.

▸ Keep your feet dry. You may not think about drying your feet off when you get out of the shower — especially between your toes. But if you're prone to athlete's foot, this is a must.

▸ Wear socks, and change them often. Keep in mind, fungi thrive in damp sneakers. Socks absorb moisture, and you can change them when needed.

▸ Get the right socks. Experts often suggest you slip into socks made of synthetic fiber that "wicks" moisture away from your feet faster than cotton or wool.

▸ Cover cuts and scrapes. Open wounds are an open invitation to all kinds of germs.

Athlete's foot can attack at any age, but if you treat your feet right, you can be ready for sandal season all year long.

Do It Better

Shoe secrets give fungus the boot

Fungus loves warm, sweaty sneakers more than a millennial loves Starbucks. The good news is you can kill those sneaker-loving germs with a shining solution — UV light.

You'll find ultraviolet light sanitizers online. Just slip them into your shoes, and relax while they kill fungus and reduce odor. The downside is they may not kill 100 percent of the bad guys, and they can be pricey.

Want to try other options first? Follow these footwear tips to keep athlete's foot at bay.

- Don't wear the same shoes every day. Let them dry out between wears, so you're not breeding bacteria and fungus.

- Let your feet breathe. Ventilated sneakers, open-toe shoes, and sandals allow moisture to escape.

- Toss tight shoes. Snug pumps may trap moisture and cause friction, which can irritate your skin even more.

Wipe out athlete's foot with 5 natural healers

Treat feet with a "fragrant" kitchen staple. Can you believe one of the greatest medical discoveries — the world's first antibiotic — started with a piece of moldy bread? It's true.

Alexander Fleming put penicillin on the radar in 1928 when he discovered a bacteria-killing mold on some old bread. Since then, it has become the cream of the crop for fighting bacterial infections.

Unfortunately, this antibiotic won't do anything for fungal conditions. The good news is you can find a natural antibiotic in your kitchen that's as strong as penicillin, but also fights off fungus.

Garlic's nickname, "Russian penicillin," says it all. Scientists think its antifungal abilities come from a compound called ajoene. In fact, a small study found that 1 percent ajoene cream applied two times a day was just as good at treating athlete's foot as Lamisil, a popular antifungal cream.

You won't find ajoene gels or creams in your local store, but some experts say you can get the benefits by adding crushed garlic to a foot bath and soaking for 30 minutes. If you prefer a salve, mix minced garlic with olive oil, and rub it on your foot with a cotton ball.

Soothe toes and soles with an essential oil. When your feet are itchy, burning, and inflamed, you'll do anything to ease the pain. Luckily, you can turn to a natural oil that beats your biggest symptoms, and then some.

Infection-fighting tea tree oil may clear up athlete's foot completely, says one study. That's what happened for more than half of participants who slathered either a 25 percent or 50 percent tea tree oil solution on their feet for four weeks.

Before you dive in, test a small spot on your healthy skin. Some people have skin reactions, but if the spot stays clear, you're good to go. Rub tea tree oil on your feet three times a day, and don't forget the area between your toes. Keep doing this for at least a week after the rash is gone to make sure you really nip it in the bud.

When you buy tea tree oil at a local health food store, open the vial and make sure you can smell a strong, eucalyptus-like medicinal scent. This is a good indication the oil contains enough of the active ingredient.

Refresh feet with a household favorite. It's strong enough to kill bacteria, yet safe enough to eat. Vinegar is a real multitasker. You can use it to clean countertops, freshen up the fridge, and even get rid of sneaky symptoms that can make athlete's foot worse.

▶ The acid in vinegar banishes bacteria that could find its way into your foot through blisters and cracks and cause further infection. Vinegar also helps fight the fungus itself.

▶ At the same time, the acid cuts through odors, acting as a deodorizer to neutralize stinky feet.

To take advantage of vinegar's healing powers, mix one cup of vinegar with four cups of water, and soak your feet for 10 to 15 minutes once or twice a day.

Cornstarch wicks away moisture for dry, happy feet. Warm, moist toes are the ultimate playground for athlete's foot. To make them a little less friendly to fungus, sprinkle clean feet with a little cornstarch. It absorbs extra moisture, which may prevent fungus from taking root and sticking around.

And here's a hot tip — brown the cornstarch in the oven before putting it to work. That will remove extra water from the powder, allowing it to soak up more moisture from your feet. Simply put the cornstarch on a baking sheet, and bake it at 325 degrees for a few minutes until lightly brown.

Calm your skin with a salty blend. Epsom salt's reputation for easing aches, pains, and stress started way back in Shakespeare's day. Maybe if Macbeth had used this remedy, he wouldn't have been so cranky. While his story ends in tragedy, your brush with foot fungus doesn't have to.

In fact, one of the lesser known benefits of Epsom salt is relieving the agony of athlete's foot. How? Epsom salt is not actually a salt. It's a combination of magnesium and sulfate. According to the Epsom Salt Council, these nutrients can reduce swelling, soften skin, eliminate odors, and draw out infections.

To score the benefits, use Epsom salt at least three times a week. Dissolve a half cup into a gallon of lukewarm water, and soak your feet for 15 minutes. Now say "Ahh."

Back pain

"It's bad news when you get to the age where your back goes out more than you do," quips popular cartoon character Auntie Acid. But it's no laughing matter if you're among the 80 percent of Americans who battle debilitating back pain. And once you've had one painful episode, you're likely to experience another within a year. What can you do?

Start with the basics. What's causing it? It could simply be the stress and strain of everyday activities. The telltale grab in your back when you bend over to weed the flower bed. That sharp stab when you reach a little too high to snag a fly while playing baseball with the kids.

But sometimes you can't pinpoint the cause, especially if your symptoms began gradually. Maybe you lifted something incorrectly or twisted the wrong way while walking, sitting, or even sleeping. Good home care — including heat, ice, and over-the-counter medicines — will usually help this type of back pain disappear within a few weeks.

Sometimes your back hurts because your spine, muscles, disks, and nerves aren't working together the way they should. This may result in acute pain that can be successfully treated with medication or exercise.

But for about 20 percent of back sufferers, acute low back pain can develop into chronic pain that may not respond to treatment. If so, your doctor will look for underlying conditions like these.

Disk problems. The shock-absorbing disks that cushion the bones of your spine may be wearing down. The soft material of the ruptured or bulging disk could be pressing on a nerve, causing your pain.

Arthritis. Osteoarthritis is the most common form to affect your back. The cartilage that cushions the bones breaks down, causing the bones to rub together. They can also form spurs that press on nerves.

Spinal stenosis. Arthritis can cause the space around your spinal cord to narrow, putting pressure on your nerve roots. You feel a tingling, weakness, numbness, or pain radiating from your lower back and down your legs.

Osteoporosis. The bones in your back can develop painful stress fractures as they become more porous and brittle.

So what are the chances you'll develop back pain? Check out these risk factors.

▸ You're overweight, underactive, and over the age of 30. A middle-age trifecta.

▸ Your DNA could be responsible. Researchers know that some forms of arthritic back pain, for example, can be caused by heredity. Thanks, Mom and Dad.

▸ Sitting at a desk all day can be rough on your back. So can a job that involves a lot of lifting. Do it wrong, and your back will let you know.

▸ And then there's smoking. You know it contributes to cancer and heart disease, but you may be surprised to learn it plays a role in back pain. Smoking may actually block healing nutrients from getting to the disks in your back. Smokers tend to heal more slowly, too, so it takes longer for you to recover.

Read on to learn about some practical ways you can make your back pain back off.

8 gentle remedies for low back pain

Rise and shine the right way. Be nice to your back in the morning, and get out of bed slowly. First roll onto your side. Bend both knees, and push yourself up with your hands. Then swing your legs over the side of the bed, and push off with your arms. Don't bend forward at the waist to get up or you could strain your back.

Relaxing your body helps mend your back. Researchers were surprised to find that stress reduction techniques were as effective in dealing with pain as behavioral therapy or a combination of drugs and physical therapy.

A study published in *The Journal of the American Medical Association* reported that 342 volunteers with low back pain took part in a program that taught them how to use relaxation techniques to manage chronic pain. After 26 weeks, almost half of the volunteers who used the training reported their back pain had significantly improved.

You can find information on relaxation techniques online or at your local library or bookstore.

Gentle stretching helps tune your spine. Lie on your back on the floor with your knees bent, your feet flat on the floor, and your hands behind your head. Point your elbows toward the ceiling while keeping your shoulders flat on the floor. Slowly lower your elbows toward the floor, stopping when your arms feel tight. Hold the stretch for 30 seconds, and then return. Repeat two to four times.

Trade your Tylenol for Aleve to beat those back blues. Emergency rooms treat more than 2.5 million back-pain sufferers every year. And their go-to medications are NSAIDs like Aleve or Advil, and acetaminophen like Tylenol, combined with opioids and muscle relaxants.

Before you pop all those pills, think about this. A recent study of over 300 people with low back pain showed NSAIDs alone were just as effective for pain relief as combinations of oxycodone, acetaminophen, and cyclobenzaphrine. Researchers also found that people who took Tylenol for their back pain stood a higher chance of developing liver problems.

So stick with plain ibuprofen to relieve your pain. If it bothers your stomach, you can switch to acetaminophen, but don't take more than 3,250 milligrams a day.

Soothe your back with a warm bath. Ahhh. Add these fragrant oils to your bath, and enjoy a relaxing soak that will calm those back spasms. Combine 1 to 2 teaspoons of your favorite carrier oil with a dozen drops of lavender and rosemary essential oils. Pour the mixture into your bath, and soak for 15 to 20 minutes. Just remember the oil may make the tub slippery, so be careful when getting out.

Rub out back pain with nature's healers. Treat your sore back to a little heat — the kind nature packed into spicy hot peppers. Look for over-the-counter rubs and ointments that contain capsaicin, an organic compound that gives chili peppers their zing.

To get the full benefit of capsaicin, apply a thin layer of the cream to your skin every day. Use a cotton ball or gloves to protect your hands. Don't be surprised if you feel some warmth, burning, or stinging as the capsaicin starts to work. And don't get discouraged if it doesn't help right away. You may have to wait up to two months for capsaicin to do its job.

> Capsaicin works by blocking substance P, a chemical that transmits pain signals to your brain.

Want a natural healer with a little less zing? Try arnica, which comes from a yellow-orange flower that grows in the mountains of Europe and Siberia. It's been soothing aches and pains for more than 400 years.

Arnica-based creams and ointments can be effective in treating sore muscles and inflammation, so it may be just what you need for your back.

Try a "heavenly" herbal remedy. Devil's claw may not sound heavenly, but it may provide glorious relief when it comes to lower back pain.

Although not well-known in the United States, the herb is used widely in Europe to treat headaches, arthritis, and back pain. One study has found it may relieve low back pain as well as a prescription drug.

Look for a supplement that will give you at least 50 milligrams (mg) of harpagoside a day, the herb's active painkilling ingredient.

Avoid devil's claw if you have ulcers or gallstones or take a blood thinner, as the combination could increase your risk of bleeding. Pregnant and nursing women should also steer clear of this herb.

Calm your aching back with ginger. You know it's great for treating your queasy stomach, but did you know ginger has also been used for centuries to treat inflammation and sore muscles? Ginger contains gingerol, an anti-inflammatory ingredient that can work wonders on your painful back — from the inside.

For a comforting cup of ginger tea, simmer fresh ginger root slices in hot water for 30 minutes, and pour the fragrant liquid into your favorite cup. Relax and enjoy.

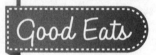

Keep your ginger fresh and tasty

To get the most from your ginger, buy it fresh — not powdered — and store it in your refrigerator for up to three weeks.

Can't quite put your finger on how to store ginger? Here are some helpful suggestions. Wrap it in a paper towel, put it in a paper bag, or simply toss it unwrapped in the vegetable crisper.

For long-term storage, pop your ginger in the freezer for up to six months. Either put the whole root in a plastic freezer bag, or cut it into smaller chunks so you have ready-to-use portions. As a bonus, frozen ginger is easier to grate than fresh ginger.

Surprising reasons your back pain won't go away

You've lost the extra weight around your middle. You've learned to lift heavy objects the right way. You're exercising regularly, and you've even given up smoking. But your back still aches. So what gives?

Your feet are in bad shape. Pain in your feet can throw your whole body off kilter. A subtle limp caused by sore feet can alter your gait and cause you to strain your back. The treatment is straightforward — fix your feet, relieve your back.

You're wearing worn-out shoes. Speaking of feet, take a look at those shoes you're wearing. They may be your favorites, but the soles are worn down, causing strain on your feet and back. Comfortable shoes that fit correctly might just be the ticket to get you back on a pain-free track.

Depression and pain go hand in hand. Chronic pain can wear you down and affect your mood, leading to depression. But it may work the other way as well.

A new study out of Australia shows that people with symptoms of depression are 60 percent more likely to suffer low back pain. Scientists aren't sure why, but one theory is that depressed people are less active and have problems sleeping, which can lead to back pain.

Antidepressants, pain management programs, therapy, and stress reduction techniques can help treat both problems so you get back to normal faster.

You're spending too much time on your phone. An active social life is important to fight off depression. But continually looking down to text or dial your phone could add an extra 60 pounds of pressure on your neck and spine, experts say. That's like carrying around a 7-year-old child all day long. Ouch.

So be aware of your posture. Let your eyes look down to check your Twitter feed while you keep your head up and your back straight.

An overstuffed wallet or oversized purse can jack up your pain. Gentlemen, if you carry that bulging wallet in your back pocket, you might be injuring your back. When you sit, your wallet could be pressing on your sciatic nerve, causing you lots of pain. Solution? Try carrying your wallet in a jacket pocket, or simply take it out when seated.

Ladies, take a good look at that bulky pocketbook you sling over your shoulder every day. Try weighing your handbag on your bathroom scale. Shocked by all the extra weight you're lugging around? See if you can slim the contents down to a manageable 2 or 3 pounds. Your back will thank you.

Constipation could be the culprit. Irregular bowel movements cause wastes to build up in your large intestine. This irritation can inflame your back muscles, causing even more pain.

Straining on the toilet aggravates the situation, too. Constant pushing puts extra pressure on the disks in your spine, making them bulge and causing you terrible pain. Don't let this happen to you. Drink lots of water, get plenty of exercise, and fill your dinner plate with fruits, vegetables, and other high-fiber foods. If dietary changes don't help, try using a fiber supplement regularly.

You're a gum chewer. Studies show that too much jaw move-ment — like when you're chewing a mouthful of Doublemint — can stress the jaw joint and cause tightness all along the back and spine.

Do you have trouble opening your mouth wide? Does your jaw click or stick? Do you grind your teeth? All signs of jaw problems. Leave the Bazooka for the grandkids, and suck on a peppermint instead.

Secret to a stronger, pain-free back (and flatter belly!)

When Brad's skiing skills started to suffer, he knew it was time to get help for his sciatica. The pain was making it difficult for him to handle even the most basic turns. Sure he was getting older, but he certainly wasn't ready to give up his favorite winter sport. Then he tried one exercise — the side plank — that relieved his pain and got him back in slalom shape, ready to hit the slopes.

A strong core is key to a strong back. Exercises that strengthen your core muscles keep your hips, pelvis, lower back, and abdomen working together so you can stand straight and tall — and pain-free.

While a weak core can lead to lower back pain and muscle injuries, a strong core increases your flexibility, balance, and stability. That makes it easier for you to complete your daily activities, from tying your shoes to skiing the slopes.

Pilates, yoga, and dancing are just a few of the fun ways to get your core back on track. But if you're looking for one exercise that takes just seconds a day, will flatten a bulging belly, and strengthen your back — with no sit-ups required — try the side plank.

Planking offers proven results. Scoliosis — a sideways curving of the spine — usually develops in children. But a combination of aging and a breakdown of the spine, possibly due to osteoporosis, puts adults at risk as well. You may have developed scoliosis and not even know it. But the side plank can help.

In a seven-month study of people with scoliosis researchers noted that the painful curvatures showed marked improvement when participants performed the side plank. Doing the exercise on a regular schedule made all the difference, though. People who practiced it for at least 90 seconds, four times each week, showed the most improvement — up to almost 50 percent.

The side plank has been successful in treating other kinds of back pain, too. Like Brad's sciatica. But you've got to stick with it to see results.

Choose a position that works for you. If you find the classic side plank too difficult, try a modified version. For extra support, position yourself close to a wall.

If you can't get down on the floor, try the simple version on your bed. Just be aware it will be more unstable than the floor, says one physical therapist. She says you should only use the bed to do a simple side plank where you keep your legs and hips down and lift your upper body.

Don't forget to check with your doctor before attempting this exercise.

Classic side plank. Lie on your left side with your legs extended. Push up and straighten your left arm. Extend your right arm straight up, using the wall for support if needed. Raise your hips so your body is in a straight line from shoulders to ankles.

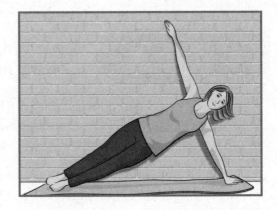

Contract your stomach and leg muscles. Hold the position as long as possible, working up to 90 seconds. *Repeat, lying on right side, left arm extended.*

Modified side plank. Lie on your left side resting on your elbow. Extend your right arm straight up, using the wall for support. Raise your hips off the floor, keeping your shoulders, hips, and ankles in a straight line. *Repeat, lying on right side.*

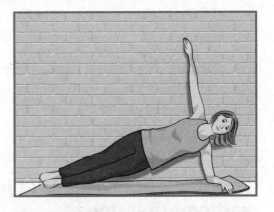

Simple side plank. If raising your hips is too difficult, follow the directions for the modified side plank, but rest your legs and hips on the floor, lifting only your upper body.

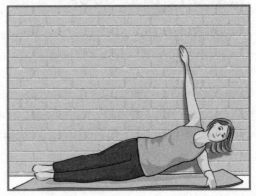

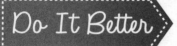 **A good night's sleep puts back pain to rest**

Nearly two out of three people with back pain also have trouble sleeping, which can make back pain worse. Knock out your sleep problems with these tips.

- Avoid afternoon naps. A little afternoon shuteye might seem like a good idea, but it could disrupt your sleep-wake cycle, making it even harder to get a full night's rest.

- Drink some cherry juice an hour before bed. Or snack on a handful of these tasty sweet treats instead. Tart cherries are chock full of melatonin, a hormone that tells your body to go to sleep.

- Wake up at the same time every day. A regular routine helps set your circadian rhythm, aka your body clock. You'll be ready to hit the hay — and fall asleep — right on schedule every night.

Popular treatments that just don't work — and one that does

Research has shown that some treatments for back pain won't do you much good. Here are some of the most common.

Bed rest. Too much bed rest can actually make your back pain worse and may even lead to complications like blood clots in your legs, loss of muscle tone, and depression. The best advice?

Begin stretching exercises as soon as you can, and try to get back to your normal routine as quickly as possible.

Traction. This common treatment is supposed to pull your spine into alignment by using weights and pulleys. While you may get some temporary relief, there is no proof that traction provides a long-term cure.

Shoe insoles, orthotics, or back belts. These devices just don't do the job, according to a study published in *JAMA Internal Medicine*. In fact, researchers found that back pain sufferers who used them were more likely to face another bout of back problems within a year.

What works? Keep active. Researchers found that exercising — along with learning better lifestyle habits — reduces your chance of another back attack in the next year by almost half. And it doesn't matter what kind of exercise you choose provided you don't overextend or twist suddenly. Lunges, stretching with possible overextension, and sports involving contact or twisting could aggravate a back injury.

You can work on your core and back muscles or go with strength training, balance exercises, walking, or an aerobic routine. The key to success? Just get moving.

To get you started, try this body roll first thing in the morning — even before you get out of bed. Lie on your back with your legs straight. Stretch your arms out over your head. Use your core muscles to roll to your left and onto your stomach. Don't cheat by using your head, arms, or legs.

Roll back onto your backside, then use the same technique to roll to your right. Gradually work yourself up to 10 reps.

Ready for more core-building challenges? Try these plank variations

You don't need hours at the gym to build a strong core. You can even do this exercise while relaxing by the pool in your favorite lounge chair.

Sit on the floor with a wedge-shaped pillow or other item that supports your back at a 30-degree angle to the floor. If you pre-fer not to sit on the floor, recline on a chaise lounge with the back tilted to a 30-degree angle. Keep your legs straight in front of you and your arms bent at the elbows with your hands placed behind your head. Press into your heels and lift up your hips to form a straight line from your chest to your feet. Hold for as long as possible.

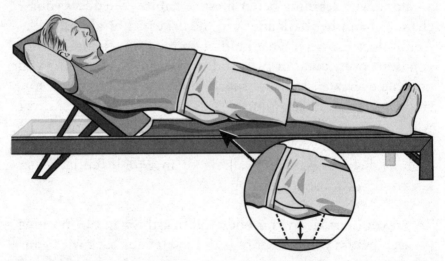

You can also flip over and perform the move lying face down on the floor. Place your hands under your shoulders, and flex your feet so you're on your toes. Raise your hips slightly and contract the muscles in your abdomen, buttocks, and legs. Hold the posi-tion as long as you can.

Blisters

Has this happened to you? You buy a new pair of shoes and can't wait to wear them, only to have them rub your feet raw with blisters. Ouch!

Those aggravating little bubbles form when your hands or feet repeatedly rub up against something — like the handle of a shovel or tight-fitting loafers. But, surprisingly, you can also get them from allergies, infections, or a nasty sunburn. Even medications can trigger blisters.

Some blisters fill with blood, aptly called blood blisters. But most fill with a clear liquid called serum, which leaks in from nearby tissues. This liquid protects the area underneath so it can form new skin. That's one of the reasons you shouldn't pop a blister — you could expose that new skin to infection.

So be patient and give your blister time to heal. Your skin will eventually reabsorb the liquid and return to normal. If the blister does pop, wash it with soap and water, and protect it with an antibiotic ointment and a bandage.

Call your doctor if a blister is really big and painful or if you develop a fever. Also watch for signs of infection like redness, extra pain and swelling, and pus.

Otherwise, you can soothe those irritating blisters with natural remedies that you may already have at home.

9 ways to take the 'ouch' out of blisters

Make sure it's well protected. Whoever invented the adhesive bandage was a genius! These stretchy, sticky little marvels will protect an entire host of skin irritations, including blisters.

Place a bandage loosely over the blister so you have a little "breathing room" between the padding and the top of your blister. This will keep your blister dirt-free while it heals.

Mix coconut with chamomile for a soothing salve. Heat 2 tablespoons coconut oil with 1/3 to 1/2 cup olive oil on low. When the coconut oil melts, remove it from the heat and let it cool for a few minutes. Add about two dozen drops of chamomile essential oil. Stir and pour into a jelly jar or small mason jar.

After the salve cools, massage it on your blister and cover with a bandage. Reapply as needed. Seal your jar and store in a cool, dry place.

Pamper your blister with petroleum jelly. Sometimes all your blister needs is a little break from friction to start healing. Petroleum jelly can help. Dab on a little and reapply as needed so you don't continue to rub it raw. This wonder balm creates a protective seal, locking in moisture while allowing your skin to heal.

Soothe your pain with heavenly oils. Nothing smells more soothing than the scent of lavender. Not only does this essential oil calm your mind, it also soothes your skin. Combine it with myrrh essential oil, and you've got a match made in heaven.

Add a few drops of myrrh and lavender essential oils to two cups of water. Next, apply one drop of each essential oil directly

on your blister followed by a drop of olive oil. Skip this part if
the blister has broken.

Place a clean washcloth in the lavender-myrrh solution, wring it,
and place it on the blister for about 10 minutes. Dry the area
and cover with a bandage.

Special salt provides quick healing. Soaking your wound in
salt may help. But don't reach for the table salt. You'll need
Epsom salt, a mineral compound that's not actually salt but a
combination of magnesium and sulfate.

Epsom salt has been used for centuries to relieve pain and muscle
cramps as well as ease stress and anxiety. Its other benefits
include soothing skin irritations like blisters.

If your blister has popped, soak it in Epsom salt to help draw
out the liquid. After soaking, dry the area and put a fresh bandage on it until the skin heals.

Treat it with germ-fighting tea tree oil. Because of its antibacterial properties, tea tree essential oil is the perfect remedy for a
nagging blister. Soak a small cloth in ice cold water, then sprinkle it with a few drops of tea tree oil. Apply it to your
blister for up to five minutes.

Not only will it protect your blister from infection, it will work
as an astringent, helping it to dry out and heal faster.

Another way to enjoy tea tree's healing properties, especially if the
blister has popped, is to add a dozen drops to four or five cups of
cool water. Soak your blister for 15 to 20 minutes, then gently dry
it. Repeat a couple of times a day until the blister heals.

Enjoy the coolness of aloe vera gel. Sometimes a blister feels like a burn. That's when you snip off a piece of aloe vera plant and massage the soothing gel onto your blister. Or you can pick up a bottle of aloe vera gel at your local drug store or herb shop.

Aloe is a natural skin healer and anti-inflammatory. Once a blister bursts, aloe will minimize swelling and hydrate the new skin, allowing it to heal faster.

Add green tea to battle inflammation. No, drinking tea will not make your blister go away. But using it topically might. Green tea combined with baking soda fights germs and inflammation when applied to your skin.

Bring several cups of water to a boil, and toss in a few green tea bags. Give the tea time to brew, then mix in a teaspoon of baking soda.

Wait for the liquid to cool, then soak your blister. Or apply the tea to your blister with a clean cloth.

Blend oils to make a calming balm. Warm up about 1/3 to 1/2 cup coconut oil on low heat until it melts. Stir in 6 to 8 teaspoons of calendula oil and remove from heat. Allow the mixture to cool for a few minutes, then stir in up to 20 drops of lavender oil. Pour into a jelly jar.

Once it cools, apply this fragrant balm to your blister for soothing relief. Repeat as needed. Remember to seal the jar tightly and store in a cool, dry location.

Easy (and cheap!) way to prevent blisters

It may be the No. 1 way to prevent blisters, and it costs only a few dollars at your local drugstore.

Paper tape applied to runners' feet before a huge race kept blisters at bay in most cases, shows a study published in the *Clinical Journal of Sport Medicine*.

Researchers followed 128 runners, all participants in a 155-mile, global ultramarathon. They applied tape to blister-prone areas on the runners' feet. They also left other areas of their feet untaped. After seven days of racing, three-quarters of the runners were blissfully blister-free in the areas the tape was applied.

Also called surgical tape, paper tape is not as sticky as bandages and other adhesives, so it doesn't pull and tear at the blister. It's also cheap and easy to use. Simply apply in single strips to blister-prone spots.

So if the fear of blisters keeps you from running, or kicking up your heels on the dance floor, no more excuses. A little tape is all you need.

Breast cancer

Merry developed a painful lump on her left breast in 2012. Most breast cancer tumors don't cause pain, so she wasn't worried and neither was her doctor. But this lump grew bigger and more painful over several months. After another visit with her doctor, he ordered a mammogram, ultrasound, and biopsy. They revealed what no woman wants to hear — she had advanced-stage breast cancer.

"It was millimeters away from becoming metastasized," says the vibrant piano teacher. Thankfully, it was caught just in time and she has lived to tell about it.

Merry is one of the 2.8 million breast cancer survivors in the United States. Even though it's the second-leading cause of cancer-related death in women (after lung cancer), there's hope for the future. Fewer women have been dying of breast cancer since 1989, thanks to better awareness and screening.

In fact, only one in 36 women, or about 3 percent, die from the disease. That means if you get it, your chances of survival are pretty high.

So how do you know if you're at risk? For one thing, you may have inherited traits that would make breast cancer more likely to develop. Surprisingly, your height makes a difference. A recent German study reported that taller people are at higher risk of developing breast cancer. Other genetic factors include your gender and the health of you and your family.

For instance, if you're a woman over 55 with a family history of breast cancer, you're at much higher risk than a younger woman with no history of the disease. And if your dad or brother had prostate cancer, your risk of breast cancer goes up as well. The two cancers seem to cluster in families, researchers say.

Living with diabetes? A Canadian study shows you're more likely to develop advanced-stage breast cancer compared to those without diabetes.

While some things are out of your control, you can still fight to overcome your risk factors and stay healthy. Along with following the tips in this chapter, you should quit smoking, and talk to your doctor about risks if you're on hormone therapy.

Also, keep those mammogram appointments. Mammography catches breast cancer in 84 percent of women, according to the Susan G. Komen Foundation.

And Merry, who's been cancer-free for several years, makes one other suggestion. "I think women need to be more aware of their bodies' changes and talk to their doctors when something seems off," she says. "I'd rather be a hypochondriac than dead."

6 habits to cut breast cancer risk

Focus on cutting calories and eating healthy foods. Eating low-carb, low-calorie meals two days a week and Mediterranean-style dishes five days a week could protect you from breast cancer, say British researchers. They found that a group of women who followed a healthy version of the popular 5:2 diet experienced changes in breast tissue that may ward off cancer.

Some studies have linked high sugar intake to a higher risk of breast cancer. When you deprive your body of calories two days a week, you have less sugar going into your cells. Restricting calories may also help you lose weight, another good way to lower cancer risk, experts say.

If you cut calories two days a week, then you should eat a healthy Mediterranean diet on the other five days, the researchers recommend. These meals, brimming with fish, fruit, herbs, whole grains, olive oil, and vegetables, arm your body with antioxidants and natural anti-inflammatories. These are vital to the fight against breast cancer.

If you're at risk for breast cancer and want to try this 5:2 diet, talk to your doctor to see if it will be helpful for you.

Go green and become a cancer-fighting machine. Eating leafy green vegetables is one sure-fire way to battle disease. But of all the nutrients found in greens like kale, spinach, and turnip greens, one stands out the most for breast cancer prevention — lutein.

Lutein is a carotenoid best known for protecting against age-related macular degeneration. You may be familiar with other carotenoids like beta carotene, found in carrots and cantaloupe. They are natural plant pigments that work as super antioxidants.

Recent studies show a connection between lutein and a lower risk of certain types of breast cancers. Lutein seems to work by blocking cancer cells from forming. The same is true of carotenoids found in red, yellow, and orange fruits and vegetables.

You can't beat eating a rainbow of colorful veggies to battle breast cancer, especially leafy greens. So follow Popeye's advice and eat your spinach.

'C' if you're getting too much of this vitamin

If you already eat plenty of grapefruit, oranges, and bell peppers, good for you. You're filling your body with cancer-fighting vitamin C. But if you take a vitamin C supplement as well, you may be doing yourself more harm than good.

Vitamin C is chock-full of antioxidants that scavenge cancer-causing free radicals and block cancer cells from forming. But you don't want to overdo it. A recent study published in the *American Journal of Clinical Nutrition* found a higher risk of breast cancer in postmenopausal women who ate foods high in vitamin C and took a C supplement to boot.

Scientists say they need to do more research to understand why. To be on the safe side, continue eating your favorite vitamin-C foods, and leave the supplements at the store.

Brush away cancer risk with healthy gums. Brushing and flossing may do more than maintain the health of your teeth and gums. Surprisingly, they could lower your chances of getting breast cancer, too.

Postmenopausal women with periodontal disease (PD) are at higher risk of getting breast cancer over those with a clean bill of oral health, say scientists who looked at data from more than 73,000 women. They also found that women with PD who smoked had an even higher risk of cancer — even if they quit smoking within the previous 20 years.

Periodontal disease develops when your gums become infected with bacteria and start swelling and bleeding. Previous studies have shown a link between PD and other chronic diseases. But scientists have only recently discovered harmful oral bacteria in breast cancer cells.

Practice good oral hygiene daily and visit your dentist about every six months. As the comedian Soupy Sales once said, "Be true to your teeth and they won't be false to you."

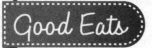

What you should eat to block breast cancer (it's yummier than you think!)

If you're looking for foods that lower your chances of getting breast cancer, look no further. This menu is based on cancer research.

Start with a salad of kale and other leafy greens, and top with chopped walnuts. Drizzle with a dressing made with extra virgin olive oil.

For your entrée, prepare a savory piece of fatty fish, like salmon or tuna. Just don't flame-broil it because that creates chemicals that raise your cancer risk.

Enjoy a side of brown rice sprinkled with flaxseeds, the tiny, tasty seeds that kill cancer cells dead in their tracks. Plus, steam a colorful array of veggies like broccoli, carrots, and winter squash.

For dessert, reach for a sweet piece of fruit.

All of these foods are brimming with phytonutrients like beta carotene, or omega-3 fatty acids. They're just what you need to arm yourself against breast cancer.

Limit protein until you reach 65. Protein does a lot of important jobs in your body. Too bad it can't cut your cancer risk — or can it? Turns out it depends on your age. It seems this powerful nutrient doesn't lower cancer risk when you are young — but it cuts cancer rates in half when you're a senior.

People between 50 and 65 years of age who ate a high-protein diet were four times more likely to die from cancer over the next 18 years, a study showed. Even a moderate-protein diet raised their cancer death risk threefold. In fact, some researchers say eating animal protein is almost as bad for your health as smoking.

But there's a silver lining. People who ate mostly plant proteins did not suffer those high cancer rates. And for those over age 65, eating a moderate-to-high-protein diet reversed their likelihood of dying from cancer by a whopping 60 percent.

Experts say older people need more protein to stay healthy because their aging bodies don't absorb or process it as well. But when you're younger, eating too much protein can raise levels of insulin-like growth factor (IGF), a hormone that regulates cell growth. And that can lead to cancer.

Exercise gives breast cancer a run for the money. Is your body on idle most of the day? Then it's time to get moving, because exercise gives breast cancer a knockout punch.

Researchers found that leisure-time physical activity reduced breast cancer risk when they examined studies involving 1.4 million people between the ages of 19 and 98.

They think it's because exercise affects your metabolism and hormones in such a way that it stunts cancer cell growth. Being active also lowers inflammation, boosts your immune system, and helps antioxidants fight off harmful free radicals.

The average amount of exercise was 150 minutes a week, or about 30 minutes five days a week.

An analysis of another 38 studies involving over 4 million women drew the same conclusion. Vigorous exercise for four to seven hours a week slashed breast cancer risk by 31 percent, say French researchers.

These scientists think it's because exercise lowers the number of fat cells that produce estrogen, a breast cancer trigger. Only women who had taken hormone replacement therapy did not benefit from exercise.

And if exercising helps you maintain a healthy weight, that's even better. Postmenopausal women who are obese or overweight raise their breast cancer risk by 17 to 58 percent, experts say. The heavier you are, the greater the risk. Another good reason to maintain a healthy weight throughout your life.

Think twice about that party drink. You enjoy a glass of wine with dinner or an occasional margarita with the girls. What's the harm in that? Probably more than you think.

Alcohol is a carcinogen, which means it causes cancer. That's what experts say, and it's a hard truth to swallow.

Multiple studies show drinking raises your breast cancer risk, even if you're just a light drinker. One study found just one alcoholic drink a day raises your chances of getting breast cancer. And the more you drink, the higher the risk.

The number of women affected by alcohol worldwide is astonishing. Researchers blame alcohol for 144,000 breast cancer cases and 38,000 related deaths in one year alone.

It's hard to imagine that a few drinks could wreak that much havoc on your body. But here's what alcohol does.

▸ changes hormone levels

▸ creates carcinogens when your body metabolizes it

▸ interferes with certain metabolic pathways that would normally protect you from cancer

▸ promotes the BRAF cancer-causing gene

▸ mimics and boosts estrogen activity, which raises breast cancer risk

Sobering, isn't it? And yet you've probably heard alcohol has some redeeming qualities, especially when it comes to your heart. Studies show light to moderate drinking — like a little wine with dinner — does have cardiovascular benefits. But experts warn the heart benefits may not outweigh the cancer risk, especially if you have a family history.

Win the battle against 2 serious side effects

If you're dealing with chemotherapy to treat your breast cancer, side effects like constant fatigue and hair loss can be devastating. But there is hope. These two new approaches may give you some much-needed relief.

"Cool" way to hang on to your hair. Chemotherapy attacks cells that divide quickly. That's good for those fast-growing cancer cells. But not so good for hair cells. They divide rapidly, too, and the chemicals attacking the cells don't know the difference.

Now there's an FDA-approved device to help you keep your hair as you go through breast cancer treatment. A "cold cap" is basically a scalp-cooling accessory worn before, during, and after chemo sessions.

Cold caps work by lowering your scalp's temperature, making hair cells divide more slowly so they're more likely to resist chemo, say scientists. They may also work by constricting blood vessels, which limits the amount of chemo that reaches hair follicles.

Most women who use them keep at least half their hair. Some experience only a mild thinning of the hair on their head, although they do lose hair elsewhere on their body.

Check with your doctor to see if cold cap treatment is available in your location.

Natural way to rejuvenate. A traditional Chinese practice shows promise for relieving fatigue, even a year after chemo. Acupressure — not to be confused with acupuncture — uses firm pressure instead of needles to stimulate points on the body. And you can learn acupressure yourself and do it at home.

More than six out of 10 breast cancer survivors who received acupressure for six weeks felt less tired compared to those who were not treated with acupressure, shows a study published in *JAMA Oncology*.

The women were taught to apply one of two types of acupressure — relaxing or stimulating. Both helped with weariness, but the women who used relaxing acupressure also reported better sleep and an improved quality of life.

Researchers say acupressure is easy to learn and could be a low-cost way to manage fatigue. They're working on an app so you can learn acupressure from the convenience of your smartphone or tablet.

Amazing tests offer hope for the future

New!

Hope. It's the one word every woman wants to hear when faced with breast cancer. And it's what new blood tests may offer in the near future.

Danish scientists studied blood samples looking for changes in metabolic patterns — changes that occur prior to any physical evidence of cancer. Knowing this may help doctors predict if you'll get breast cancer within the next five years, they say.

"The method is better than mammography, which can only be used when the disease has already occurred," says researcher Rasmus Bro. "It is not perfect, but it is truly amazing that we can predict breast cancer years into the future."

Swedish scientists looked at blood samples to see if they could predict whether breast cancer would metastasize, or spread to other parts of the body.

First they studied tumor samples with genetic changes. Then they explored blood samples looking for identical genetic changes. Women with genetic mutations in their blood were eventually diagnosed with new tumors. The women with clear blood samples were not.

The researchers hope their findings will help doctors detect the spread of tumors much earlier, giving patients a higher chance of survival.

Bruises

It's been decades since Kenickie slicked back his hair and warned, "You're cruisin' for a bruisin,'" in "Grease." And while you're never cruisin' for one, you probably still find yourself sporting a colorful injury from time to time. Where do those mysterious bruises come from?

First of all, two things happen as you age that can mean more bruises.

▶ Your skin gets thinner and loses the fatty layers that once protected those small, delicate blood vessels, called capillaries.

▶ You're more likely to take medications, like aspirin or anticoagulants, and supplements, like fish oil or ginkgo, that thin your blood and lower its ability to clot.

That means when you blunder into the coffee table or smack your shin on the dishwasher, you start a chain reaction. The blow damages your muscle fibers and the connective tissue below your skin. Then blood from crushed capillaries leaks out into your skin and gets trapped, forming a pool that looks blue, black, red, or purple. Finally, the area starts to swell. Over the next two weeks, you'll notice your bruise changing colors as your body reabsorbs the trapped blood.

Unfortunately, this process can take longer as you age. So to help speed the healing, place an ice pack on the area for 20 minutes the first couple of days after the injury. Cold slows your blood flow, reducing the amount that leaks out of your capillaries, and also helps with the pain and swelling. If you elevate the bruised area above your heart, you'll also have less blood pooling at the injury site.

Here are a few other ways to ease a bruise and help it heal quickly.

5 soothing ways to heal a bruise

Embrace aloe's healing powers. Herbalists have touted the aloe vera plant's medicinal benefits for centuries, using the clear gel from its leaves to treat everything from acne and eczema to poison oak and poison ivy rashes. Supposedly, even Cleopatra smoothed it on as part of her regular skin care routine.

If you apply aloe gel directly onto a bruise, the natural healing compounds in it, called anthraquinones, will begin to do their work, repairing tissue and relieving pain.

Invest in a plant so you have access to aloe year-round. Or pick up a bottle of aloe vera gel at your local drug store or herb shop for just a few dollars.

Tap into St. John's divine relief. You probably think of St. John's wort as an antidepressant. But the plant's flowers and buds produce an oil jam-packed with antibacterial and anti-inflammatory agents, making it a natural remedy for skin irritations — including bruises.

Look for bottles of St. John's wort oil at any herb shop or order it online. Then massage it in every day until your bruise disappears.

Practice bruise control with an easy-to-make balm. Your first aid kit is probably chock-full of bandages, ointments, and antiseptics. But it needs one more thing — this bruise-healing balm, made with arnica, that can soothe the pain and swelling associated with most skin injuries.

Use low heat to warm up about a cup of olive oil and 2 tablespoons grated beeswax. Stir until the beeswax has melted completely. Allow the mixture to cool, then add 2 dozen drops of arnica essential oil. Pour into a mason jar, seal, and store away from heat and light. Apply just a bit of this fragrant balm gently to your bruise two or three times a day.

Warning

Bruised and battered: know when to call the doc

Most of the time a bruise disappears after two or three weeks and you can go on your merry way. But on occasion, a bruise means there's something more serious going on. Here are seven warning signs. If you experience any of these, pay your doctor a visit.

- You've started bruising often and for unknown reasons.

- You notice more bruising after starting a new medication.

- A bruise continues to swell and is very painful.

- A bruise is on your back, face, or trunk, or it's near your eye and is affecting your vision.

- You have a history of bleeding a lot, especially during surgery.

- Your family has a history of bruising or bleeding significantly.

- You can't move a joint near a bruise.

Essential oils say bye-bye to bruising. They are all the rage right now, but natural practitioners have been using essential oils for years to treat a variety of ailments. The following recipe speeds up bruise healing by narrowing your capillaries, which limits the amount of blood around the injury.

Mix together two to three drops each of lavender and helichrysum essential oils. Lightly massage directly onto your bruise. You may not be familiar with helichrysum, but it's a member of the sunflower family, and the oil is often referred to as Immortelle.

Want even more healing? Add a few drops of cypress, lemongrass, and geranium essential oils to your blend. Apply two to three times a day until your bruise goes away.

Put together a powerful poultice. Some call it "bunny's ear" and some call it "flannel leaf." No matter what you call it, the herb commonly known as mullein is a bruise's best friend, perhaps because of its anti-inflammatory properties.

Add a small amount of boiling water to some shredded mullein leaves — just enough to make a paste. Fold the mixture into a soft cloth, like flannel, and when it's cooled enough to handle, apply to your bruise.

Depending on where you live, you may have mullein growing nearby. But if you don't, you can order 4 ounces of dried leaves for under $4 from online herb shops.

Bug bites

Spiders and skeeters and flies, oh my! They're everywhere, making themselves right at home in your kitchen cabinets and living room baseboards. What's a person to do?

First, rest easy. Not all bugs pose a threat. Some help you by eating other bugs, like the busy rove beetle that swoops around your garden, feeding on flies, fleas, and mosquitoes.

Most bugs that live indoors are tiny and often go unnoticed. You probably don't realize your home welcomes about 100 species of insects every day. While most are fairly harmless, those that feed on live hosts can pose a threat.

A tick is one example. If it bites an animal that carries a blood-borne disease then attaches itself to you, you'll be injected with the disease. Some diseases, like Lyme and Rocky Mountain spotted fever, can be quite harmful and even deadly.

The threat of being infected by a mosquito is also scary, though not as alarming as people think. For example, most people who test positive for Zika experience no symptoms or just mild ones. Severe symptoms or death related to the Zika virus is low, says the Centers for Disease Control and Prevention.

That said, you still want to take precautions. If you plan to be outdoors and don't want to coat yourself with repellent, wear long pants and a long-sleeve shirt, and tuck pant legs into socks and your shirt into your pants. Don't wear tight clothing since mosquitoes can bite through fabric, and avoid wearing dark clothes.

As they say, the best defense is a good offense. You won't have to treat yourself for painful bites and stings if you keep the bugs away in the first place. Here are some other simple steps to ward off bugs, mosquitoes, bees, and more.

Simple steps to repel 5 pesky pests

Stamp out skeeters in a rain barrel. You hate them. Fish love them. So why not feed mosquitoes to some goldfish or a school of minnows? It's easy if you have a do-it-yourself (DIY) rain barrel.

Some rain barrels come with a solid cover, which helps to keep mosquitoes out. But many DIY rain barrels call for a mesh cover. The screen keeps debris out, but not mosquitoes. Since the stagnant water just sits there until it's needed, it's the perfect place for mosquito larvae.

That's where your fish friends come in. Goldfish and minnows love to snack on larvae. The more larvae they eat, the fewer mosquitoes you have buzzing around your yard. It's a win-win!

Look online or check your local home improvement store for affordable DIY rain barrels.

Aromatic ways to repel ticks. Natural practitioners swear by essential oils for a variety of ailments. They also use them to deter ticks.

Make a spray with rose geranium oil and/or red cedar oil. Mix 15 drops of either or both in an 8-ounce spray bottle filled halfway with witch hazel and the other half with distilled water. Shake and spray on.

Herbalists say the oils work by masking your natural body odors, making it harder for ticks to find you.

Fragrant herb makes flies fly away. You love adding basil to your pesto and pasta sauce. Here's another reason to love basil — it's a natural fly deterrent.

Place pots of the sweet-smelling herb around doorways and windows to keep houseflies out. Or sprinkle dried basil into small pouches and tie them with ribbon. Rub the little sacks periodically to release the basil's aroma.

If you're ever around horseflies, make this natural repellent. In a spray bottle, mix 2 cups vinegar with 1/4 cup baby oil and a squirt of dishwashing detergent. Shake and spray on yourself before heading out to an area with lots of horseflies.

Citrus juice sends spiders packing. Spiders hang out at your house year-round. Thankfully, limes and lemons are available year-round, too. Pour pure lime or lemon juice into a spray bottle with some water. Spray the solution around your door frames and window sills, and use to clean your countertops (except granite and marble). Not only will spiders stay away, your house will smell nice and clean, too.

Banish bees with herbs and spices. Garlic, cinnamon, and peppermint — three very different flavors with one thing in common. Bees hate them.

Make a spray adding a few squirts of dishwashing soap to water. Add either cinnamon, crushed garlic, or peppermint oil to the solution, and spray it around your house. Or better yet, place pots of peppermint on your porch or patio.

To rid your pool or garden fountain of honeybees, mix 1/4 cup dishwashing soap with about a quart of water in a spray bottle. Spray the bees directly while they're buzzing around near the water. They will die in an environmentally friendly way. When they don't return to their colony, the rest of the bees won't know where to find the water source.

What really works against mosquitoes

Victoria's Secret has a "secret" that may surprise you. Douse yourself with its perfume Bombshell, and you can kiss bothersome mosquitoes goodbye!

A recent study discovered that the perfume works almost as effectively as the repellent DEET. Instead of attracting mosquitoes, as researchers expected, the fragrance repelled the insects for over two hours. They think it's because Bombshell masks natural body odors, which attract mosquitoes.

You'll need more than a light spritz, though. Try these other products for proven-to-work protection.

Defeat bugs with DEET. Deet has long been the king of bug repellents, but many people are concerned about harmful side effects. Products containing between 7 percent and 30 percent DEET seem to be the safest and most effective, say scientists. Anything higher than 30 percent can trigger health problems like skin irritations and seizures. And anything below 7 percent won't protect you for very long.

Put on pretreated apparel. Clothing manufacturers like Burlington make shirts and pants pretreated with the insecticide permethrin. The chemical works by killing mosquitoes when they land on you or by keeping them away from you. You would still need to treat exposed skin, including face and hands, and any untreated clothing.

Another option is to buy a can of permethrin and spray on your outdoor wear. The insecticide remains effective after several washings.

Spray on semi-natural substitutes. Sprays containing 20 percent picaridin or 30 percent oil of lemon eucalyptus performed as well as DEET in a *Consumer Reports* test. Picaridin contains compounds similar to the piperine found in black pepper. The gum eucalyptus tree produces oil of lemon eucalyptus. Both products have less serious side effects than DEET.

Is Avon's Skin So Soft legit? Some people swear by it, but does it really work? Yes, but only if you use the right product. Both Skin So Soft Bath Oil and Skin So Soft Bug Guard offer protection, but they work on different types of mosquitoes.

In one study, the bath oil protected against the *Aedes aegypti* variety but was ineffective against *Aedes albopictus*. The bug guard had the opposite results. If you're a fan of Skin So Soft products, you may want to experiment to see which works best in your neighborhood.

Canker sores

It started as a tingling sensation on the inside of your lip, and now it's a painful, open sore. Professionals call it an aphthous ulcer, but you know it as the dreaded canker sore.

Cankers are not cold sores. Many people confuse canker sores with cold sores, also called fever blisters. Those painful blisters, caused by the herpes virus, appear on the outside of your mouth. Canker sores typically pop up inside your mouth. They love the soft inner surface of your cheeks, lips, tongue, gums, and the back of the roof of your mouth.

Cankers appear as white spots surrounded by a red border of inflamed skin. While they're not contagious like cold sores, they can be just as painful.

Hidden triggers to watch out for. Scientists aren't sure what causes mouth ulcers. They suspect sores may be triggered by hormonal changes, stress, injury to your mouth, or problems with your immune system. It may even be your diet. You may see more of them pop up if you're low in certain vitamins and minerals, particularly iron, folic acid, and vitamin B12.

Canker sores generally go away on their own. But in the meantime, you have to deal with the ouch factor when you try to eat or carry on a conversation. Pain often goes away within a week, but it can take a few weeks for a canker sore to completely heal.

Follow this advice to soothe the pain, shorten the time the ulcer hangs around, and prevent canker sores from returning.

4 tips to take the edge off canker sores

Protect your mouth with a creamy treat. Legend has it that yogurt was originally created by accident. But it's no fluke that tons of folks recommend it as a delicious defense against canker sores.

Yogurt is chock-full of probiotics — good bacteria that keep the bad guys in check. They help restore the balance of bacteria in your gut. And they do the same for your mouth.

Some studies have suggested that imbalances in mouth bacteria may contribute to recurrent sores. One study out of Korea found that the probiotic *S. salivarius*, in particular, helped decrease the risk of mouth lesions. Experts also say *L. acidophilus* and *L. bulgaricus* may help people with recurrent canker sores.

Look for all these probiotics in the ingredients list of your favorite yogurt. And be sure it says "Live & Active Cultures" to get the most benefit.

As an added bonus, this marvelous-for-your-mouth treat may also fight bad breath and keep your teeth strong and your gums healthy.

Heal your sores with a sticky (but sweet) remedy. Honey has been hailed as a wound healer for ages. So it makes sense it can heal a tiny wound in your mouth. It even has research to back it up.

Scientists divided 94 participants into three groups and asked each group to apply a different treatment to their canker sores — commercial honey, a steroid cream called triamcinolone, or the pain reliever paste Orabase.

Honey reduced the pain, size, and redness of cankers faster than the specially formulated products. This sticky soother could heal your sore in just three days. Sweet.

Soothe cankers with a quick rinse. They call them sores for a reason, but if you get hit with painful cankers, you don't have to grin and bear it. Swish with one of these homemade mouthwashes for one minute to soothe the pain.

▸ Rinse with a mixture of half hydrogen peroxide and half water. Be careful not to swallow.

▸ Swish with a cocktail of half Milk of Magnesia and half Benadryl liquid allergy medicine.

▸ Add some salt to a glass of warm water, and gargle to soothe your sore.

▸ Brew a cup of chamomile tea, let it cool, and swish it around your mouth. You can even put the cooled tea bag right on the sore to reduce irritation.

▸ Mix one cup of warm water with a half teaspoon of powdered licorice root. Use a tablespoon of the mixture for each treatment. Regular licorice root can raise blood pressure, so make sure you get deglycyrrhizinated licorice (DGL).

Avoid triggers you can control. A good way to prevent painful cankers is to avoid things that may trigger sores or make them worse.

▸ Watch out for foods that irritate your mouth. Pay special attention to sharp foods like chips and toast, spices like cinnamon and salt, and acidic fruits such as pineapple and oranges.

▸ Be gentle with your mouth. Don't brush too vigorously. Cut out bad habits like chewing your lip.

▸ Avoid toothpastes and mouth rinses that contain sodium lauryl sulfate. This ingredient may provoke canker sores in some people.

Cold lasers — a hot topic for canker treatment

New!

One canker sore can make you cranky, but when they become repeat offenders, you may feel positively helpless. Luckily, a new therapy is delivering results.

Low-level laser therapy (LLLT), also known as "cold laser," uses light to stimulate tissue cells and fight inflammation. Studies show it may speed up healing time, relieve pain, and reduce the size of sores in people with minor recurring cankers. It may also put a stop to frequent outbreaks.

While the treatment option needs further study, the future for canker sufferers looks a lot less gloomy.

Colds

It's called "common" for a reason. Everybody gets one now and then. In fact, Americans suffer through 1 billion colds annually — more than any other illness. They are the reason for almost 100 million doctor visits each year, and they cost the economy more than $20 billion in lost work days.

The common cold is actually a viral infection that takes over your upper respiratory tract, irritating your nose and throat. More than 200 types of viruses can cause your illness, but the rhinovirus is the worst offender.

And you certainly recognize those symptoms. Runny nose, hacking cough, aches, and pains. They may seem common to everyone else, but when you've got them, they're anything but ordinary. In his poem, "Common Cold," Ogden Nash wrote, "Bacteria as large as mice, with feet of fire and heads of ice, who never interrupt for slumber, their stamping elephantine rumba." A pretty eloquent way to describe the misery that comes with a sore throat, sneezing, fever, and congestion.

Sure, you try to protect yourself. You wash your hands umpteen times daily, avoid those coughing coworkers, even pump up your vitamin C. But still one of those 200 viruses attaches itself to the lining of your nose or throat, and you know a cold is brewing. How did it happen?

Maybe you handled a surface that had germs on it, like a doorknob, remote control, or computer keyboard. Then you touched your mouth or nose. Gotcha. Or perhaps you got too close to someone who was already infected, and they coughed or sneezed into the air. You breathed in the virus and — 10 to 12 hours later — your symptoms began. Now you're dancing your own "elephantine rhumba."

What can you do to relieve your worst cold symptoms? Read on for some tried-and-true cold comforters.

Breaking news from the cold front

New!

This is nothing to sneeze about. Scientists think they've finally figured out how to make a vaccine that will protect you from the common cold.

Until recently, this seemed like a pharmaceutical pipe dream, because the most common cold-causing virus, the rhinovirus, has more than 100 strains. Creating a vaccine for each and every type seemed an impossible task.

So researchers tried a different approach. They took 50 types of rhinovirus and mixed them together into one vaccine. They wanted to see if the human immune system could make antiviral antibodies to protect against each strain. And so far, it's worked — in the lab.

More research is needed, but it may not be long before you'll be lining up to get that long-awaited, cold-curing shot in the arm. A true medical marvel.

6 ways to fight your cold war — and win

Honey-sweet remedies clobber your cold symptoms. Rid yourself of the misery of even your worst cold. All you need is a little honey plus some of your favorite foods, and you'll be feeling better in no time.

▸ **Honey, and — coffee?** Who knew this duo could fight off cold symptoms? But a three-year study showed a combination of coffee and honey significantly eased chronic coughing. Simply stir together 3/4 cup honey and 1/2 cup instant coffee crystals until it forms a thick paste. Three times a day for one week, measure 1 tablespoon of this mixture into 7 ounces of warm water, mix, and drink. The caffeine will relax and widen the major air passages in your lungs, while the honey is, itself, a cough suppressant.

> Honey is the perfect alternative to harsh prescription cough syrups. For example, your doctor may have prescribed Tussionex, an antihistamine, narcotic cough suppressant combo. Be careful. If not taken correctly, Tussionex can cause life-threatening side effects. Make sure you're getting the correct dose by using a marked measuring spoon or syringe — not a regular tablespoon.

▸ **Honey and tea.** For a delicious three-in-one remedy that soothes a sore throat, stops a cough, and helps you sleep, stir a little honey into a steaming cup of chamomile tea. The honey will calm your cough and ease sore throat pain, while the chamomile will help you relax for a good night's sleep.

▸ **Honey and pineapple.** Pineapple contains bromelain, a natural substance that helps reduce mucus. Paired with honey, this combination provides soothing relief from your cough. Try mixing a little honey into a cool glass of pineapple juice, or drizzle a teaspoon over pineapple chunks for an all-natural remedy.

Breathe easier with a common spice that will really fire things up. Cook with cayenne pepper and you just might ease your latest cold or flu symptom. Sprinkle a little into your favorite soup or stew, and you'll feel this friendly fire go to work on your chest congestion, cough, and stuffy nose.

Cayenne works by thinning the mucus in your nasal passageways, making it easier for you to breathe. And the pepper even warms your body from the inside out, relieving those uncomfortable chills. If you can tolerate adding sliced chili peppers to your favorite recipes, you'll also get a massive dose of vitamin C, another popular remedy for battling the common cold.

Spice things up with a cayenne pepper "tea" you can sip all day long. Pour 1 cup boiling water over 1/2 teaspoon of cayenne powder. Stir to combine. Measure out a teaspoon of this solution and add to a glass of water. Drink up to four times every day as needed to relieve your symptoms.

Battle your cold with steam power. Put a stop to coughs and congestion with vapor treatments using healing oils.

▸ **Tea tree and eucalyptus.** Known for their antiseptic and antiviral properties, these two oils help relieve your sinus congestion and stuffy nose. Make a soothing vapor by combining five drops each of eucalyptus and tea tree oils in a heat-resistant bowl. You can adjust the amount of oil according to your preference. Next, pour in several cups of boiling water. Don't get close enough to burn your skin, but lean over the bowl, carefully draping a towel over your head to trap in the fragrant steam. Take deep breaths through your nose for several minutes. Do this two or three times every day.

▶ **Camphor.** This aromatic vapor will clear your chest congestion, soothe your cough, and help you relax. In a shallow container, combine 1 1/2 cups hot water with one drop camphor essential oil. Sit in a comfortable position and lean your head over the bowl. Using a towel to tent your head and the bowl, breathe deeply for at least three minutes. Lift the towel for fresh air as needed. Repeat this treatment daily for best results.

To keep colds at bay, spice up your life. You sprinkle it on your morning oatmeal, add a dash to applesauce, enjoy it on a baked sweet potato. But did you know your old standby spice — cinnamon — can stave off cold viruses?

"A diet that includes a tablespoon of cinnamon once or twice a day can be effective in eliminating or preventing viruses from infecting humans and causing sickness, such as colds and flu," says Dr. Milton Schiffenbauer, a microbiologist and deputy chair of the biology department at the New York School of Career and Applied Studies (NYSCAS).

Schiffenbauer's team tested Saigon and Ceylon cinnamon, and found both fight off a specific virus similar to one that infects people. If that's not enough, the spice is packed with antioxidants, which can boost your immune system and get you back on your feet in no time.

Soothe even your worst cold with these two aromatic teas.

▶ Simmer two cinnamon sticks and some sliced fresh ginger in water for 20 minutes. Strain and enjoy.

▶ Drop a cinnamon stick into boiling water. Continue boiling for two minutes, and then remove the stick. Use the cinnamon water to make your favorite herbal tea, like good-for-you green tea. Drink twice a day to ease your cold symptoms.

Sage advice for sore throats. Whether it's fresh from your garden, or dried in a jar, sage provides soothing relief for your irritated throat by slowing the development of bacteria and drying up mucus. And when you combine sage with apple cider vinegar and salt — two well-known natural healers — you create a powerful antibacterial pain-relief remedy.

▶ Measure 2 tablespoons of dried sage, or 4 tablespoons fresh, into the bottom of a small bowl. Pour 1/2 cup boiling water over the leaves. Cover the bowl, and steep for 15 minutes.

▶ Meanwhile, pour 1/2 cup of apple cider vinegar into a glass jar, and sprinkle in 1/2 teaspoon salt.

▶ Strain the sage tea, and add the liquid to your vinegar salt solution.

▶ Gargle a mouthful of the mixture three times a day.

Close your jar up with a tight-fitting lid, and store the remaining liquid in the refrigerator for up to one week.

Dip your spoon in a super bowl. To relieve your cold symptoms, reach for some plain, simple, comfort in a bowl — chicken soup.

Sure it's an old-fashioned cure that's been around for ages, but modern science has provided up-to-date proof that it really works.

White blood cells called neutrophils are ready and waiting to protect your body from infections. But researchers think these cells can become over-active and increase inflammation, causing many of the symptoms you experience during a cold. Chicken soup, packed with vegetables, herbs, and rich broth, has anti-inflammatory properties that curb the neutrophils and give you a fighting chance at beating the infection.

> Want even more cold-fighting power? Drink two cups of cranberry juice every day. Experts think the colorful natural compounds in cranberries help fight infection from cold and flu by strengthening your front-line immune cells so you experience fewer symptoms. Plus, it improves memory and keeps your blood sugar steady.

It's not just Grandma's homemade recipe that touts these "souper powers," either. Studies show a combination of ingredients in chicken soup — whether it's store-bought, homemade, or even canned — work together to bring you symptom relief. Soup also keeps you hydrated, provides healthy nutrients, and wraps you in warm, steamy comfort. Heat up a bowl and enjoy.

Is the internet making you sick?

Only half of all Americans were connected to the internet a few years ago. Today the number of users has exploded to more than 80 percent of the U.S. population. Unfortunately, this Wi-Fi frenzy may have created a health problem no one predicted.

Researchers studied 500 people, ages 18 to 101, who spent an average of six hours online every day. The group with the most screen time reported 30 percent more cold symptoms than less frequent internet users.

That same group reported being stressed when they were disconnected from the web, but felt relief when they reconnected. This cycle of stress and relief caused their levels of cortisol — a hormone that affects the immune system — to rise and fall, putting them at greater risk of catching a cold.

Bottom line? Power down your screens to power up a healthier immune system.

Missed your flu shot?
Vitamin D to the rescue!

Who Knew?

It's easy to forget about getting a flu shot — until you come face-to-face with someone who has a case of influenza. But don't worry. Vitamin D may be all you need to keep from getting sick.

Most flu outbreaks happen in the winter when people aren't getting much vitamin D from the sun. Researchers don't think that's a coincidence. Vitamin D actually boosts your immune system and helps you fight off infections like the flu. One way it does this is by amping up natural antibiotics in your body that wipe out invading germs.

To make up for those short winter days, eat more vitamin D foods like salmon, sardines, mushrooms, and fortified cereals and milk. Or take a supplement of at least 600 international units (IU) a day.

Colon cancer

Would you believe colon cancer is one of the most preventable types of cancer? In fact, experts say you can reduce your risk by 50 percent if you just follow these simple cancer-prevention guidelines.

Live a healthy lifestyle. Start by making four important changes.

▶ **Eat smart.** This means avoiding saturated fats, red meat, processed meats, and highly processed carbs like sugary sodas. Scientists say the heme iron in red meat can damage your colon's lining and trigger cancer-causing substances. Plus, sugar seems to feed cancer cells, and leads to weight gain and glucose imbalances, both of which raise cancer risk.

▶ **Get moving.** Studies show the more active you are, the more you're protected from colon cancer. Make exercise part of your daily routine by shooting for 30 to 60 minutes of moderate to vigorous activity.

▶ **Drink less.** The more alcohol you drink, the higher your colon cancer risk. The ethanol in alcohol naturally breaks down into a toxic chemical that can damage your DNA, increasing your cancer risk. Plus it creates harmful oxygen-containing molecules, called free radicals, that wreak havoc throughout your body.

▶ **Maintain a healthy weight.** Your waist size is strongly related to your risk for a number of cancers, including colon cancer. Scientists suggest it has something to do with the high levels of insulin you have in your body when you're overweight or obese.

While you can't do much about a family history of cancer, you can stack the odds in your favor by not smoking and working with your doctor to control certain diseases like diabetes, Crohn's disease, and ulcerative colitis that increase your risk of developing colon cancer.

Get regular screenings. No one likes to get a colonoscopy, but this routine screening may save your life. Colon cancer rates have dropped 30 percent over the past two decades in adults 50 and older. Researchers believe it's because more people are getting screened. Colonoscopies enable doctors to find and remove pre-cancerous polyps. Plus, treatment is more successful when colon cancer is detected early.

Don't ignore these symptoms. Sometimes your body is trying to tell you something. While it doesn't necessarily mean you have colon cancer, see your doctor if you suddenly experience:

▸ diarrhea or constipation.

▸ bloody or narrow stools.

▸ frequent gas, cramps, bloating, or fullness.

▸ unexplained weight loss.

▸ pain or tenderness in your lower abdomen.

11 foods that kick colon cancer to the curb

The great diet swap — how fiber can save your life. Here's an easy equation. A diet high in fiber but low in fat and protein equals a slashed risk of colon cancer. And here's the proof.

A team of British and American scientists asked a group of rural South Africans to swap their high-fiber diets for a Western diet. Think burgers and fries, spaghetti and meatballs, and sausage biscuits. Guess what happened? Their colon cancer markers spiked after just two weeks.

At the same time, a group of African Americans switched up their Western diet for a typical South African menu — one loaded with fiber but low in fat and protein. For two weeks they munched on corn fritters, mango slices, lentils, navy bean soup, and fish tacos. The results were astounding — less colon inflammation and lower cancer risk markers.

It all comes down to your gut bacteria, known as your microbiome. The bacteria that live and thrive here help digest food, destroy organisms that cause disease, metabolize drugs, prevent infection, and provide you with nutrients. A diet that's high in fiber nourishes the good bacteria in your microbiome. And that, in turn, promotes a healthier colon.

In this case, more fiber triggered the production of butyrate, a robust cancer-fighting substance.

The small study has prompted researchers to explore prevention and treatment therapies that target gut bacteria. In the meantime, there's no reason you can't add more fiber to your diet, starting today.

▸ Eat fruit like apples and pears with the skin on.

▸ Enjoy legumes like baked beans and lima beans.

▸ Graze on greens like spinach and broccoli.

▸ Toss nuts and seeds on your salad instead of croutons.

▸ Cook with whole grains like barley and oatmeal, and choose whole-wheat bread.

Reel in real protection with fatty fish. Are you a pescovegetarian? A what, you say? Don't be offended. You are one if you eat only vegetables — that's the "vegetarian" part — with some fish and seafood thrown in for variety — that's the "pesco" part. This type of diet is also called pescatarianism, and if you eat this way, you are really giving colon cancer a one-two punch.

Vegetarians already have an advantage over meat-eaters when it comes to colon cancer, with all the natural plant nutrients in their diet. But a study published in the highly acclaimed journal *JAMA Internal Medicine* showed when veggie-eaters ate fish at least once a month, they slashed their colon cancer risk even more. In fact, pescovegetarians had the lowest colon cancer risk in the study.

Even more amazing, if you've been diagnosed with colon cancer, a little fatty fish on the menu could boost your chances of survival, since research shows it can kill cancerous cells and shrink tumors.

Scientists say it's the omega-3 fatty acids in fish that make it a powerhouse against colon cancer. On top of that, this natural nutrient also fights high blood pressure, osteoporosis, and Alzheimer's disease.

You'll get a megadose of omega-3 from fish like mackerel, salmon, and herring, but there's a good amount in certain plants, too. Here are a few ideas you should try:

▸ Sprinkle flaxseeds or chia seeds on your breakfast cereal.

▸ Snack on a handful of walnuts.

▸ Cook with canola or soybean oil.

The amazing apple — your new ally against cancer. Lady Alice, Granny Smith, and Aurora — sounds like the cast of "Downton Abbey," doesn't it? But these are actually varieties of one of the best cancer-fighting fruits around, the apple.

It doesn't seem to matter if you eat them fresh or dried, or drink the juice — apples knock out cancer with a powerful punch. You can thank polyphenols, nutrients that annihilate cancer cells before they take root. One study out of Italy showed eating a medium-sized apple a day lowered the risk of colon cancer by 30 percent. Other studies suggest drinking apple juice reduces colon cancer markers.

Plus, eating apples may help you live longer. Why? Because this humble fruit also battles heart disease, high blood pressure, high cholesterol, and Alzheimer's. How 'bout them apples!

Punch out cancer risk by the bunch. Say *gracias* the next time you meet a Spaniard. Their ancestors brought grapes to America about 300 years ago. Little did they know those tasty orbs were packed with powerful cancer-fighting compounds.

One of them, resveratrol, is a potent antioxidant found primarily in grape skins. The best news — it stops the cancer process dead in its tracks.

One study, in particular, showed eating a third of a pound to a pound of red, seedless grapes a day for two weeks blocked events on a cellular level that lead to colon cancer. People over 50 showed the most benefit.

Grapes are also rich in other healthy nutrients like anthocyanins, catechins, and quercetin. So it's really no surprise this one fruit fights high blood pressure, high cholesterol, and diabetes, along with cancer. Munching on grapes even cuts your risk of dementia by over 75 percent. *¡Muy bien!*

Spice up your fight against colon cancer. This deadly disease doesn't stand a chance against one delicious food. Can you guess what it is? Surprise, it's curry. The magic begins with the Indian spice turmeric. It contains curcumin, which researchers say acts as an anti-inflammatory and curbs the formation and growth of cancer cells.

In addition to canceling out colon cancer, curcumin also battles cancers of the breast, lungs, skin, prostate, pancreas, and more.

If you're not fond of the taste of curry, try this tip that adds the benefit of curcumin to your diet without any hassle. Pick up a jar of ground turmeric at your local supermarket, and sprinkle it on eggs, green beans, and other veggies. Or add turmeric to your mashed potatoes. It will turn them a golden yellow, without any detectable taste difference.

Great news for coffee lovers. Been wondering if you should give up your coffee habit? Unless your doctor tells you to stop, keep on guzzling.

Drink one to two servings of coffee a day and you could slash your risk of colon cancer by 26 percent, say University of Southern California researchers. Go back for thirds — or even more — and your risk is cut in half.

You may want to drink a lot of strong coffee if you're fighting colon cancer. A large study out of the Dana-Farber Cancer Institute found people with stage III colon cancer were less likely to have their cancer return after treatment if they drank at least four cups of caffeinated coffee every day.

Both caffeinated and decaf seem to work, so it's not the caffeine. Plus, espresso, instant, and filtered all serve up a heaping scoop of protection. So what's in coffee that protects you from colon cancer?

▸ Melanoidins produced during the roasting process trigger your ability to "go," moving cancer-causing substances out of your body.

▸ Diterpenes are oily compounds in coffee beans that help your body defend itself against damage from cancer-causing free radicals.

▸ Polyphenols are a group of natural chemicals in many plants that also act as antioxidants to stop the growth of colon cancer cells.

Rice and potatoes — they're better for you than you think.
Remember that low-carb phase you went through, where you swore off rice, pasta, and potatoes? It's time to put them back on the menu, say researchers. These foods are superheroes in the fight against colon cancer.

It's all thanks to a type of starch your body can't digest, dubbed "resistant starch."

Acting like fiber, resistant starch makes its way from your mouth all the way to your colon without undergoing much change. While in your colon, it ferments and becomes a prebiotic, feeding the good bacteria in your bowels. That good bacteria creates a fatty acid called butyrate — and that's what protects you from cancer. Butyrate lowers the pH level in your colon, pares down inflammation, and stops cancer cells from growing.

In fact, resistant starches are so good for you, they can cancel out the damaging effects of foods that raise cancer risk. A study published in the journal *Cancer Prevention Research* reports the number of tumor-producing molecules spiked by 30 percent in the colons of people who ate a diet high in red meat. But those who ate red meat along with resistant starches kept these cancer markers at bay.

There are three types of resistant starch you'll want to know about:

▶ The first type occurs naturally in certain foods like green, unripe bananas.

▶ The second kind forms when you cook then cool starches like rice, pasta, and potatoes. That means you can get a good dose of resistant starch from refrigerated pasta or potato salads.

▶ The third type is in seeds, grains, and legumes. Eat chick-peas and lentils, for instance, for the resistant starch making up the cell walls in these plants.

Cancer protection from the produce aisle. Hands down, the two most promising foods in colon cancer prevention are cabbage and broccoli. Here's why.

A look at 35 studies shows these two cruciferous vegetables are loaded with glucosinolates, natural compounds that protect against tumors, act as antioxidants that eliminate free radicals, and help keep normal cells from turning into cancer cells. As an added bonus they have lots of fiber, which bulks up your stool and eliminates it quickly, carrying potential cancer cells along with it.

Other glucosinolate-rich vegetables are Brussels sprouts, cauliflower, collard greens, kale, kohlrabi, mustard, rutabaga, turnips, and bok choy.

So how do you know if you're getting enough? A six-year study out of the Netherlands showed people eating 2 ounces of cruciferous vegetables a day — that's equal to about one-half cup of cabbage — were significantly less likely to develop colon cancer than those eating just a third of an ounce — or less than 2 tablespoons of cabbage. Of course, experts recommend you get at least 2 1/2 cups of vegetables a day for better overall health.

Now that you know you need to eat more broccoli and cabbage, give these two healthy recipes a try.

Recipe

- Slice a head of broccoli lengthwise into three "steaks." Coat with olive oil, sprinkle with a little salt and pepper, then toss on the grill.

- Instead of traditional, mayo-soaked slaw, try shredding a head of cabbage then mixing it with rice vinegar, grated ginger, scallions, and cilantro. Add finely chopped chili pepper for extra zing.

Wash away cancer risk with this surprising drink. Forget all those milk mustaches. What celebrities should be touting is buttermilk, the moo juice that's filled with cancer-fighting fuel.

This creamy, slightly tart beverage contains certain lipid and protein molecules that, in laboratory tests, slowed or stopped the spread of colon cancer cells. In addition, you'll get a heaping helping of good bacteria, also known as probiotics, with every sip. These "good bugs" can throw a monkey wrench into the process of forming colon tumors by:

▶ interfering with cancer-causing enzymes.

▶ preventing dangerous changes to normal cells.

▶ lowering bile acid in your colon that can make cells reproduce too fast.

▶ reducing inflammation.

▶ speeding waste out of your body so cancer-causing toxins don't have time to form.

Down a cold cup of lowfat buttermilk, and you also get 8 grams of protein, 28 percent of your daily calcium requirement, and a helping of important B vitamins. All for less than 100 calories.

To start adding buttermilk to your menu, check out these delicious tips.

▶ Substitute low-fat buttermilk for regular milk in your smoothies.

▶ Marinate homemade chicken nuggets in buttermilk for at least an hour, then coat with bread crumbs and bake.

▶ Toss avocado chunks, vinegar, and buttermilk in a blender to make a de-lish salad dressing.

▶ Whisk mayo and buttermilk with dill and caraway seeds for a tangy veggie dip. Add salt and pepper to taste.

▶ Use buttermilk instead of regular milk to make your mashed potatoes.

Aspirin therapy: homespun miracle cure?

Who Knew?

Your fight against colon cancer just got easier, thanks to a drug you already have in your medicine cabinet — the humble aspirin.

Health experts say you should consider taking a low dose of aspirin every day if:

- you are between the ages of 50 and 70.

- you can commit to taking it for at least five to 10 years.

- you don't have an increased risk of bleeding.

Their recommendation is based on research like a Danish study which shows people who took 75 to 150 milligrams of aspirin regularly for five or more years cut their risk of colon cancer by 27 percent. Doctors believe the credit goes to aspirin's anti-inflammatory properties.

But taking this popular and inexpensive pill can come with risks, which include bleeding ulcer and hemorrhagic stroke. In addition, a small percentage of people with certain genetic markers actually raise their risk of colon cancer by taking aspirin. So make sure you talk to your doctor before starting any new treatment.

Say nuts! to colon cancer. Eating healthy doesn't have to be boring. Just reach for walnuts. Their nutritional benefits tower above peanuts, pecans, pistachios, macadamias — even almonds.

Here's the proof. Mice fed a diet fortified with walnuts developed fewer colon tumors compared to those who ate none. Scientists believe it's because these little nuggets of goodness have a probiotic effect in the colon, making the environment healthy and strong against cancer.

Plus, walnuts are packed with two powerful, cancer-fighting substances — omega-3 fatty acids and vitamin E.

But they're not just a heavyweight against cancer. This "king of the nuts" combats heart disease, gallstones, diabetes, and weight gain.

So take plain pasta or brown rice and add some hearty crunchiness by tossing in a handful of walnuts. Seven a day is all it takes to reap the benefits.

Enjoy a simple snack with built-in cancer protection. Songbirds have good reason to devour those sunflower seeds in your neighbor's bird feeder. Not only are sunflower seeds rich in vitamin E and fiber, they're also a good source of selenium. Research results on selenium and cancer have been mixed, but many studies seem to agree that too little selenium can increase your cancer risk. In fact, low selenium is a problem in parts of Europe. A recent study of more than 500,000 Europeans found that women with higher selenium intakes had lower odds of getting colon cancer than women who got less.

To boost your selenium, stir sunflower seeds into trail mix, muffins, salads, or even smoothies. If you need more selenium, enjoy foods like canned light tuna, roasted turkey breast, canned sardines, and pulled pork in barbecue sauce.

Looking for trouble: 5 screening options to consider

"Screening for colorectal cancer is effective and can save your life," says Tom Frieden, Director of Centers for Disease Control and Prevention (CDC). Yet more than 20 million adults in this country haven't had their recommended screening and may end up dying from a preventable tragedy.

The truth is a colonoscopy is still the No. 1 way for doctors to find colon cancer and remove polyps. But if you can't stomach the idea of getting screened this way, here are a few alternatives for people at low risk. Just make sure your insurance covers the procedure and your doctor approves.

Name of Test	Advantages	Disadvantages	Frequency
Cologuard (Stool DNA test)	Stool sample collected at home and sent to lab • No bowel prep or diet restrictions • Stool is checked for blood and 11 colon cancer markers	A positive result means you have to get a colonoscopy anyway • Finds abnormalities when none are actually present	Every 1 to 3 years
Fecal Immuno-chemical Test (FIT)	Stool sample collected at home and sent to lab • No bowel prep or diet restrictions • Detects blood in the stool	A positive result means you have to get a colonoscopy anyway • Cannot detect some polyps or cancers	Annually
Fecal Occult Blood Test (FOBT)	Stool sample collected at home and sent to a lab • Detects blood in the stool • No bowel prep	A positive result means you have to get a colonoscopy anyway • Cannot detect some polyps or cancers	Annually
Sigmoid-oscopy	Less extensive bowel prep than traditional colon-oscopy • Polyps can be removed during the procedure	Only checks the rectum and lower third of the colon • A colonoscopy may still be required	Every 5 years
Virtual colonoscopy or CT colonography	No sedation • Can spot suspicious tissue and large polyps	A positive result means you have to get a colonoscopy anyway • Requires bowel prep • Radiation exposure	Every 5 years

Constipation

When you can't "go," your digestive system is like a train that's stuck on its tracks.

Normally there's a beginning, an end, and a few stops along the way. First, you chew your food. Then it travels down your esophagus into your stomach. From there it moves to your small intestine and on to your large intestine. Lastly, it cruises through your rectum and out of your body. Along the way, a combination of chemicals, gastric juices, and muscle contractions break everything down and move it along. That is, if the journey goes smoothly.

Sometimes, though, things happen that block the tracks. And you get constipated. Often, it's due to one of the following:

▸ not enough fiber in your diet

▸ dehydration

▸ lack of physical activity

▸ stress

▸ travel

▸ ignoring the urge to go

▸ some medications like antacids, antidepressants, or pain relievers

▸ various medical conditions including irritable bowel syndrome (IBS), diabetes, colon cancer, or thyroid problems

Everybody gets stopped up from time to time, but doctors say you have chronic constipation when you experience these symptoms regularly:

▶ You have fewer than three bowel movements a week.

▶ Your stool is hard and dry.

▶ You strain every time you go.

▶ You still feel full after you've gone to the bathroom.

All is not lost if you struggle with constipation. Just making simple lifestyle changes will help. However, if you simply can't find relief, pay your doctor a visit. It could be a sign of a more serious condition.

Warning

Surprising health risk of chronic constipation

There's a connection between your heart's health and constipation, and you're not going to like it.

People who frequently struggled to go to the bathroom were at a higher risk of dying from heart disease and stroke, found a Japanese research team.

Scientists used data from over 45,000 people, ages 40 to 79, throughout a 13-year span to draw their conclusions.

They're not saying this definitively proves constipation can cause death from heart disease. But they do suggest constipation that requires straining could raise blood pressure which increases stroke risk. Doctors suggest you avoid straining excessively if at all possible.

6 things you can do to flush out constipation

All backed up? Focus on fiber. When your doctor says, "Eat more fiber," you may hear, "Eat food that tastes like cardboard." No worries. It's very easy to find an abundance of foods that are fiber-filled AND delicious. Each will help you move things along when you need fast relief from constipation.

First, understand the basics of fiber. It's found in all plant foods, but it's the part you can't digest. There are two kinds.

▸ Soluble fiber relieves constipation by soaking up water and turning into a gel, making your stool softer and easier to move. You get it from fruit like pears, plums, apples, and berries. (See, it's not all cardboard!) Other sources of soluble fiber include foods you probably have hiding in your kitchen cupboard right now, like dried beans and oatmeal.

▸ Insoluble fiber bulks up your stool and speeds its movement through your digestive tract. You'll find it in nuts, seeds, whole grains, and vegetables like squash, green beans, celery, and cucumbers.

Many foods — like kiwifruit — have a combination of soluble and insoluble fibers. In fact, kiwi fiber contains some unique properties that really help you go, experts say. Just two kiwi a day helped people who had struggled with constipation for at least six months as well as those with constipation related to irritable bowel syndrome. Eat the fuzzy skin on your kiwi and you'll get an even bigger dose of fiber.

To make sure you're getting enough fiber, look up the number of grams on the nutrition labels of your favorite packaged foods. And remember, you can't go wrong with fresh produce. A single cup of cooked lentils has almost 16 grams (g) of fiber. A cup of raspberries contains 8 g, and a medium sweet potato has 4 g.

Do you know how many grams of fiber you should be getting?

Fiber grams per day		
Age	Women	Men
19-50	25	38
Over 50	21	30

Gut check: be proactive with probiotics. Ever wonder why so many places — from gas stations to fast-food chains — keep a stock of yogurt cups, yogurt bars, and yogurt parfaits? Maybe it's because this creamy delicious treat serves up health benefits by the billions — billions of probiotics, that is. As a form of good bacteria, they help you digest food, fight off illness, and maintain a healthy gut. Perhaps even keep you regular, since studies show probiotics make your stools softer, speed up your stool's travel time, and help you go more often.

While yogurt is a tasty way to get probiotics, you can also buy probiotic tablets, capsules, and softgels. Researchers identified the *Bifidobacterium lactis* strain as delivering the most constipation relief when they examined multiple studies. So look for that on the label.

In addition, a study out of Italy had people with chronic constipation take a tablet containing 100 million cells of the strain *Lactobacillus reuteri* twice a day, 30 minutes after eating. After four weeks, they reported going more often per week with softer stools.

Even people with constipation caused by irritable bowel syndrome (IBS) may benefit from taking probiotics or eating yogurt.

Experts now believe chronic constipation and IBS may belong to the same family of medical conditions.

Soothe your tummy troubles with essential oils. Sometimes a little TLC is all your belly needs to feel better. Especially when it's stopped up.

Try gently massaging these home remedies over your entire abdomen for five to 10 minutes several times a day.

▸ Mix a tablespoon of sweet almond oil with a few drops of orange essential oil to make a fragrant and healing mixture. Herbalists believe orange oil can treat gut problems from spasms to constipation.

▸ Combine 2 1/2 tablespoons of olive oil with five drops of peppermint essential oil, 10 drops of lemon essential oil, and 15 drops of rosemary essential oil. This combo seems to boost circulation and trigger bowel activity.

Do It Better

Potty power: squat, don't sit

The best way to go is to squat. That's why those comfort-height toilets could contribute to your constipation.

Squatting automatically relaxes your pelvic area, making it easy for you to have a bowel movement. But comfort toilets sit 2 to 3 inches higher than regular ones, which changes your sitting position.

If you have a hard time going on a taller toilet, get a foot-stool that's 7 to 8 inches high. Prop your feet on it to raise your knees above your hips.

Hands-on healing: stay regular with acupressure. Constipation relief without drugs or side effects? This remedy may sound unusual but it's effective. Simply apply a little pressure to your perineum, the area between your anus and your genitals.

Doctors think massaging here helps break up hardened stool, relax anal muscles, and trigger the nerves that help you have a bowel movement. Here's how you do it.

When you first feel the urge to go, press your middle and index fingers to your perineum. Maintain pressure until you've passed your stool.

Close to 100 people who suffered with chronic constipation learned how to perform this kind of self-acupressure, and a month later not only improved their bowel function but felt better and less stressed, found a UCLA study. Some of those in the study also drank more fluids, ate more fiber, and took laxatives or stool softeners. But those who additionally practiced perineal acupressure gained the most benefit.

Surefire way to "prune" tummy woes. There's nothing more powerful than prunes to get you going. And while you may think it's the fiber that moves things along, it may actually be something else — a natural sugar in prunes called sorbitol. Your body processes sorbitol so slowly, it has time to sit in your digestive tract, pulling in water and triggering bowel movements.

Both of these actions helped 40 chronically constipated people who ate 12 prunes a day, according to a Canadian study. They reported having an extra bowel movement a week and softer stools.

Prune juice also contains sorbitol, but the whole fruit has a higher amount.

Discover a new way to use an old folk remedy. Remember when your grandmother gulped down a shot of castor oil to relieve her "costiveness"? These days it's called constipation, and castor oil still delivers relief — just not in the way Nana used it.

Gently rub 1 to 2 tablespoons of castor oil directly on your abdomen. Then cover with an old towel, cotton T-shirt, or length of flannel fabric. Bear in mind castor oil will stain whatever you use.

Warm a heating pad to medium or fill up a hot water bottle. Wrap in another towel, place on your abdomen, and relax for about 30 minutes. The gentle heat will open up your pores and allow the castor oil to get absorbed into your body.

Rx Alert

Stop drug-induced constipation before it stops you

Four out of 10 people who take opioids like hydrocodone and oxycodone end up constipated.

It's all because these pain relievers interfere with your body's digestive process and even partially paralyze your stomach. In addition, opioids lessen your urge to go.

If you're about to start an opioid regimen, be prepared to take stimulant laxatives and stool softeners as recommended by your doctor. Don't take bulk-forming laxatives like psyllium or methylcellulose, though, as these may worsen your symptoms.

Beyond that, make sure you practice good dietary habits, like getting plenty of fiber from natural sources and drinking at least eight glasses of water every day.

Depression

Everyone has days where they feel down for no reason or struggle to get going in the morning. But if you have true depression, you feel sad almost all the time and may not even be able to get out of bed. It's a serious disease that calls for serious help from an expert. Here's how you can figure out where you stand.

You may have the blues if you:	You may be depressed if you:
have trouble concentrating when you read	have no interest in picking up a book
need convincing to go out with friends	refuse to go out at all
feel tired during the day	feel too exhausted to get out of bed
have trouble sleeping some nights	can't seem to sleep at all
continue to play in your weekly bridge game	quit most of your usual activities
feel perked up when you hear good news	take no interest in even the best news
are disappointed in some aspects of life	feel like a complete failure
feel a bit restless	feel agitated and have trouble sitting still
notice some appetite changes	have lost or gained weight for no reason
want to change certain things about life	feel trapped in your life
make some plans for the future	have thoughts of suicide

Dealing with depression isn't easy, and it's not something you can just get over. While it may not cause a fever or a cough, it's a disease just like the flu. It's caused by chemical changes in your body. Specifically, imbalances in the neurotransmitters serotonin, norepinephrine, and dopamine that control your mood. These chemicals act as messengers within your brain, so an imbalance can send the wrong message.

Factors that cause these changes can include genetics, drug or alcohol abuse, prescription medications, or other medical conditions. Chronic inflammation in your brain may trigger symptoms, too.

Older people are often at high risk, because life changes like retirement or the loss of a spouse, can also cause depression.

Being depressed affects more than just your mood. It can raise your risk of heart disease and death, and aggravate chronic conditions like diabetes, arthritis, back problems, and asthma. It may also be an early warning sign of Alzheimer's disease.

If you are depressed, you need to visit a doctor. But if you're just feeling a little blue, there are some easy steps you can take every day to boost your mood.

10 bright ideas to lift the cloud of depression

Sweat out your stress. You can't run away from your problems, but you can run away from all the stress they cause. That's because when you work out, your body releases chemicals called endorphins. These boost your mood and lower levels of the stress hormone cortisol.

But exercise is good for more than just a quick remedy. Research shows that physical activity can actually create lasting changes in your brain. A Swedish study on mice discovered that exercise boosts a special muscle enzyme that protects your brain from depression. It works by attacking a particular stress protein that can negatively affect your mood, breaking it up before it can get to your brain.

Avoid the trans fat trap. Deadly ingredients hiding in your favorite foods could raise your risk of depression. Thank goodness you can easily avoid this danger — if you know what to look for.

The hidden culprits are trans fatty acids, also called partially hydrogenated oils. Unlike other fatty acids, they don't occur naturally. Food manufacturers create them by adding hydrogen to vegetable oil. They are great for extending food's shelf life, but not so great for your health.

A Spanish study found that people who ate the most trans fats raised their risk of depression by 48 percent in just six years. Trans fats can also raise "bad" LDL cholesterol, lower "good" HDL cholesterol, and increase your risk of heart attack, stroke, and diabetes.

There are no health benefits to eating trans fats and they aren't an essential part of your diet. Fortunately, the Food and Drug Administration requires every food manufacturer to list trans fats on product labels. Remember these tips.

▶ Check the amount of trans fats on the Nutrition Facts panel of every food that has a label. Common offenders are margarine, shortening, fried foods, and junk food. Surprisingly, nutritional supplements and nutrition bars may contain trans fats, too.

▶ Beware of products labeled "trans fat free." They are legally allowed to have 0.5 grams of fat. If a "zero trans fat" product still has trans fats, you will find the phrase "partially hydrogenated" in the ingredient list.

▶ Avoid fried foods in restaurants. Many places fry in trans fats. Ask your server if a food contains trans fats or will be cooked in them, or check the restaurant website for information ahead of time.

Ditch the low-carb diet — it's making you miserable. Close your eyes and think about your favorite comfort food. Whether it's mac and cheese, lasagna, or a warm muffin, that go-to dish is probably loaded with carbohydrates.

That's because carbohydrates actually boost the amount of serotonin, a mood-regulating chemical, in your brain. In short, carbs make you happier. If you've ever tried to follow a low-carb diet, you've probably felt down and cranky. At the time, you might have thought you were just hungry, but, in reality, your brain wasn't making enough serotonin.

And worse than giving you a sour mood, a lack of serotonin is linked to mental disorders like anxiety and depression. A yearlong study found that people on a low-fat diet that allowed carbs were happier than those on carb-cutting plans, even though both groups lost the same amount of weight.

So if you're trying to trim your waistline, don't cut out carbohydrates, just try to eat healthier ones. Whole grains are a great place to start. Out of more than 72,000 women, those who ate a diet focused on whole grains, vegetables, fruits, legumes, fish, and poultry were least likely to die from any illness, especially heart disease. Plus, the type of fiber found in whole grains seems to help prevent weight gain and belly fat.

To be healthier and happier, buy the whole-grain versions of flour, bread, and pasta. A few simple substitutions mean you can eat your favorite comfort foods and still smile.

Comfort food with a twist: mood-boosting mac and cheese

For a mac and cheese recipe heavy on comfort and light on guilt, try using whole-grain elbow pasta and one of these light cheese sauces.

- Top the pasta with feta cheese and olive oil instead of cheddar and butter for a Greek twist.

- Steam then purée half a head of cauliflower. Mix with one cup of skim milk, a pound of low-fat shredded cheese, and a quarter-cup of Parmesan. Stir together with cooked pasta, pour into a casserole dish, and top with a sprinkling of bread crumbs. Bake at 350 degrees 15 to 20 minutes for a crisp, golden crust.

Snooze to lose the blues. A poor night's sleep will not only make you groggy, it can lead to depression.

Improve your mood just by improving your quality of sleep. Try these tips for a better night's rest.

▶ Stick to a regular sleep schedule.

▶ Avoid late afternoon naps.

▶ Keep your bedroom dark, quiet, and cool.

▸ Don't use your bed for anything other than sleeping and sex.

▸ Stay away from caffeine and alcohol at night.

▸ Exercise regularly, but not too close to bedtime.

Rx Alert

These drugs can bring you down

Depression can be a serious side effect of some drugs. If you take any of these and think you might be depressed, talk to your doctor immediately.

Health condition	Drug class	Drug name
pain	nonsteroidal anti-inflammatory drugs (NSAIDs)	ibuprofen (Advil), combination of acetaminophen and tramadol (Ultracet)
high blood pressure	antihypertensives	clonidine (Catapres)
heart problems	beta blockers	propranolol (Inderal)
asthma	bronchodilators	pirbuterol (Maxair)
allergic reactions, asthma	corticosteroids	prednisone
infection	antibiotics	ciprofloxacin (Cipro), gemifloxacin (Factive)
heartburn	histamine blockers	ranitidine (Zantac), cimetidine (Tagamet)

Don't worry, "B" happy. If you're not getting enough of your B vitamins, you're at risk of serious moodiness.

▶ Studies show that women with vitamin B12 deficiencies have double the risk of depression. This nutrient also affects how you think and remember, so getting enough can help keep your brain sharp. Clams, mackerel, and herring provide a megadose of this brain-boosting vitamin.

▶ Vitamin B6 produces chemicals in your brain, called neurotransmitters, that can control your mood. Fortified cereals are a great source. Just watch the sugar content.

Coffee can really perk you up. Get ready to rev up your mood. That morning joe does more than help you start your day. Studies suggest it can improve your sense of well-being and slash your risk of depression.

Researchers examining the coffee habits of 50,000 women found that those who drank two or three cups of coffee a day were 15 percent less likely to develop depression than those drinking a cup or less a week. Women who drank four cups of coffee daily cut their risk by 20 percent. Oddly enough, people who drank decaf or got their caffeine somewhere else didn't see the same benefits.

Experts aren't sure why caffeinated coffee is so effective, but they think the caffeine affects brain chemicals like serotonin, a "feel-good" neurotransmitter. Still, they need to do more research to find out what exactly makes coffee so effective.

If you're not already a coffee drinker, mental health experts don't necessarily think you should start — especially not with four cups a day. A sudden increase in caffeine can lead to nervous jitters, an upset stomach, trouble sleeping, and a rapid heartbeat. But if you already enjoy your java, scientists say two to four cups daily is safe for most adults.

Just keep in mind the researchers defined a cup of coffee as an 8-ounce beverage containing 137 milligrams of caffeine. If your brand of coffee has more caffeine or your mug is larger, you may need to adjust your servings.

To find out how much caffeine is in your coffee, check the label on the bag or can, visit the company website, or ask the barista who served you.

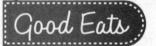

Healthy ways to blunt bitter coffee

Do you load your coffee with cream and sugar, just to cut the bitterness? If so, the calories are adding up quick. Instead, try these tricks to make a healthier, better-tasting morning brew.

- Mix one teaspoon of crushed shells from hard-boiled eggs into your coffee grounds before brewing to neutralize the acidity and mellow the flavor.

- Take your coffee off the burner within 15 minutes of brewing to keep it from getting that nasty, burnt taste. Keep it in a thermos and heat it up later in the microwave.

- Store your ground coffee in an airtight container to help the flavor last longer.

Fight the funk with omega-3 fatty acids. Experts have long suspected that cultures with high-fish diets suffer less from major depression, and people with major depression generally have low levels of omega-3 fatty acids. But now they finally have the data to prove it.

Researchers discovered that omega-3 fatty acids can improve depression symptoms just as well as prescription antidepressants. Though they are not sure what exactly makes omega-3s so effective, they have a few theories.

▸ Suffering from chronic, low-grade inflammation is a risk factor for depression. As an anti-inflammatory, omega-3 fatty acids, especially from fish oils, can lessen this risk.

▸ Polyunsaturated fats, like omega-3s, are known to control signals between neurons and influence how cells respond to specific signals. These signals often pass on information related to emotions.

▸ Not enough fatty acid in your brain could mean an imbalance of brain chemicals that influence mood.

The groundbreaking study used 1,050 milligrams (mg) of eicosapentaenoic acid (EPA) and 150 mg of docosahexaenoic acid (DHA) every day. To get these omega-3 components through your diet, eat fatty fish like bluefin tuna, Atlantic wild salmon, and herring. If you want to try supplements, make sure you talk to your doctor first.

Tune in to the healing power of music. If you have the blues, try listening to the blues. Or rock, pop, R&B, country, jazz, classical, or any other music you like. It can really beat your blahs.

In a Cleveland Clinic study, people who listened to either their favorite music or soothing tunes eased their depression symptoms by 25 percent.

But why not do more than listen? Go one step further and pick up an instrument. Researchers say playing music can fight off symptoms of stress, anxiety, and depression.

Seems it doesn't matter whether you decide to tickle the ivories, strum a guitar, or blow your horn — lose yourself in the music and you'll play the blues away.

Music not your thing? Try dabbling in watercolors or charcoal. Art therapy, an accepted treatment for mental health since the 1930s, can lift your mood, stimulate your mind, and help you relax. It can include drawing, painting, sculpting, and even discussions and interpretations of art.

Lean on your loved ones. The Beatles put it well — you can get by with a little help from your friends. Social isolation is a major contributor to depression, but having a strong support system can help you cope with life's up and downs. Do your best to stay connected to your friends and family. Get involved with local clubs and church groups.

And try to surround yourself with positive people. You can "catch" happiness from others. Studies have found that spending time with happy people will make you happier, too.

Pick up your mood with tryptophan. Whenever somebody settles in for their post-feast nap on Thanksgiving, they blame tryptophan. The amino acid does have a mild sedative effect, and it helps your body produce melatonin, the brain hormone that controls your body's internal clock.

But tryptophan can make you happier, too. After it's digested, it is converted to serotonin, a feel-good chemical that can boost your mood. Experts believe a lack of tryptophan can lead to serious mental problems like bipolar disorder and depression.

You'll find tryptophan in a lot of high-protein foods like meat, fish, turkey, and peanuts. But you'll need carbohydrates to help your brain use this amino acid. So make your leftover turkey into a sandwich and you'll be well on your way to a better mood.

Warning

Mind your meds with this natural pick-me-up

St. John's wort can be just as effective as several antidepressants for mild to moderate depression. Like some prescription drugs, the herbal remedy works by inhibiting the reuptake of serotonin, dopamine, and norepinephrine. This means that, rather than being reabsorbed and recycled by the cells that originally produced them, these chemicals remain in your brain to boost your mood.

But don't try it without asking your doctor first. The herb can weaken the power of other medications, like cholesterol-lowing drugs and blood thinners. And when it's combined with certain antidepressants, like Prozac or Zoloft, it can trigger a dangerous condition called serotonin syndrome. You might become confused, hot, sweaty, and restless, and experience headaches, stomachaches, muscle spasms, or seizures.

Seasonal depression — how you can wrestle the winter blues

If you're feeling down in the dumps during those short winter days, it might be more than the weather. You could have seasonal affective disorder, or SAD. It's a type of depression that occurs when your biological clock is out of whack, either due to bad sleep habits or lack of daylight. Here are two smart ways to cope.

Melatonin. Most people naturally cycle through periods of sleep and wakefulness that correspond to the hours of darkness and light. This cycle is regulated in part by your internal clock, which responds to signals from hormones like melatonin.

As you age, you produce less melatonin and, in the winter, a lack of daylight means your body has trouble making it properly. That's when boosting your melatonin becomes a good idea. Taking supplements at the right time of day — an hour or two before bedtime — can improve the quality of your sleep without making you feel drowsy the next morning.

You'll want to check out supplement labels before you buy melatonin. This is one case where more is not better. Massachusetts Institute of Technology (MIT) researchers found a standard dose of about 3 milligrams (mg) overloads the melatonin receptors in your brain to the point they stop working. One-tenth of that amount — or just 0.3 mg — is enough to help you fall asleep and maintain better quality sleep.

Light therapy. This involves sitting in front of a special lamp that uses multiple full-spectrum fluorescent lights. The key is this bright artificial light, measured in units called lux. Typical therapy is 2,500 lux for two hours a day or 10,000 lux for 30 minutes a day. A small study of seniors found that light therapy worked as well as antidepressants in boosting mood after just three weeks. It also helped the participants sleep better.

If you're interested, look for light boxes on the internet or in some drugstores. Just talk to your doctor first, because there are some possible side effects, like nausea, headaches, and eyestrain.

Diabetes

Diabetes is no laughing matter. It can cause blindness, nerve damage to your feet, and kidney failure — just to name a few of its debilitating side effects. This serious disease affects 12 million Americans over the age of 65, with more than a million new cases diagnosed every year. More frightening is the fact that millions of people actually suffer from diabetes but don't see a doctor for diagnosis or treatment. Could you be among them?

These are among the most common symptoms.

- frequent urination

- extreme thirst

- hunger, even though you're eating

- fatigue

- blurred vision

- slow-healing cuts or bruises

- tingling, pain, or numbness in your hands or feet

Type 1 diabetes was called juvenile diabetes for many years because it is usually diagnosed in children and young adults. It occurs when your pancreas doesn't produce insulin. You need this hormone to move blood sugar, called glucose, from your bloodstream into your cells, where it is used for energy. Only

5 percent of people with diabetes have type 1. Most learn to manage it with insulin therapy and other treatments.

Type 2 diabetes, on the other hand, is the most common type, by far. With this disease, your body actually makes enough insulin, but your cells stop using it as they should. This is called insulin resistance. Your pancreas gets the signal to make even more insulin, but the sugar levels in your blood just keep building up. You now have full-blown diabetes.

Scientists don't know exactly what causes type 2 diabetes, but they've been able to identify some risk factors. These are the ones you have no control over:

▶ Age. The older you get, the higher your risk.

▶ Race. Ethnicities at higher risk include African-American, Mexican-American, and American Indian.

▶ Family history. If someone in your family has diabetes, your chances of developing it go up.

The good news is you can lower your risk of type 2 diabetes in the first place and manage your blood glucose levels naturally if you already have it. Take a look at the factors you have some control over.

Weight. Even a little weight loss delivers big rewards. People who lost a modest 5 percent of their weight slashed

Neck size is an even better predictor of diabetes than waist size, according to a study published in the *Journal of Diabetes Research*. Experts say women with a neck circumference of 13.4 inches or less and men measuring 14.6 inches or less are not considered overweight and are therefore at lower risk.

multiple diabetes risk factors, according to a study published in the medical journal *Cell Metabolism*. That's only 12 pounds if you weigh 240.

"A 5 percent weight loss is sufficient to improve health outcomes," says Dr. Samuel Klein, senior study author, "with additional weight loss further decreasing risk factors for metabolic and cardiovascular diseases." This just shows you get a large bang for your weight-loss buck.

Diet. Make a few changes every day — like eating more fruits and vegetables and fewer chips, cookies, and soda — and you could keep diabetes at bay.

Exercise. Physical activity keeps your blood sugar steady and your heart and muscles strong while relieving stress.

10 smart ways to face down diabetes

Eat right to banish the blood sugar blues. Less meat, more produce — it's a simple formula proven to slash diabetes risk by 20 percent, according to a two-decades study published in *PLOS Medicine*. But are all plant foods created equal?

Scientists answered this question by comparing healthy choices like fruits, vegetables, whole grains, nuts, legumes, and vegetable oils, to unhealthy ones like refined grains, potatoes, and fruit juices.

Including less healthy options actually increased diabetes risk by 16 percent, while the healthier plant diet lowered risk by a whopping 34 percent. Why? Because healthy plant foods are:

▸ rich in fiber.

- needed to keep your gut bacteria healthy.

- high in antioxidants.

- loaded with vitamins and minerals.

- full of unsaturated fat.

- low in saturated fat.

All of these factors help you control your blood sugar.

Get a grip on glucose with good rice advice. It's perfect as an entrée or side dish — but only if you choose brown. Compared to white rice, which can raise your diabetes risk, nutrition experts say brown rice is a better choice because it lowers blood sugar and reduces diabetes risk. In fact, swapping out just a third of a typical daily serving of white rice with the same amount of brown rice could lower your risk of type 2 diabetes by 16 percent.

Not convinced yet? How about this. Researchers placed over-weight women on a weight-loss diet in which they alternated eating brown rice and white rice. The women lost more weight, reduced their waist size, and had better blood pressure when they ate brown.

To understand why it's healthier than white, you need to understand how rice is processed. White rice starts out as brown, but undergoes a polishing process. This removes the bran layer, which lowers the amount of fiber — and it's that fiber that keeps blood sugar levels from spiking. Polishing also raises the starch content. Generally, foods high in starch raise blood sugar levels.

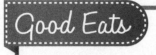
Good Eats

Great grains of goodness: a perfect way to cook brown rice

Don't shun brown rice just because you've only ever had it as a tough, gummy mess. There's a way to cook it so every grain is fluffy and perfectly cooked. Simply throw everything you know about cooking rice out the window. Instead, cook it like pasta.

Fill a large pot with plenty of water — as much as 3 quarts — and bring it to a boil. Add about a cup of long-grain brown rice, and a bit of salt, if you like. Continue boiling, stirring occasionally, for about 25 minutes. Note, this is a much shorter cooking time than the usual 50 or so minutes recommended for brown rice. You can get away with it because you're using more water. The grains move around in your pot, rather than sitting in a clump, cooking unevenly.

Now all that's left is to drain off the water and enjoy a hearty scoop.

Pick up the pace for better blood sugar. Are you discouraged by the thought of completely changing your lifestyle to avoid diabetes? Then do this one thing. Go out for a fast walk.

People who took moderately intense walks of 11 to 14 miles per week — that's less than two miles a day — lowered their blood sugar levels almost as effectively as people who combined three lifestyle changes — diet, exercise, and weight loss.

Want to count steps instead of miles? Some experts suggest a goal of 10,000 steps a day. Why not take the stairs or park your car at the far end of a parking lot. To make it easier to track your progress, get a fitness watch or app for your smartphone. Just make sure your steps are fast ones.

Vitamin D gets an A+ as a diabetes deterrent. They don't call it the sunshine vitamin for nothing. This versatile nutrient delivers a ray of hope to people diagnosed with prediabetes, a condition where your blood sugar levels are high, but not high enough to be considered full-blown diabetes. Could taking vitamin D supplements help fight prediabetes? That's the question researchers in India wanted to answer.

They found after two years, only about 11 percent of people with prediabetes who took vitamin D supplements along with 1,250 milligrams of calcium carbonate developed diabetes, compared to 27 percent of those who took only calcium. Plus, blood sugar levels returned to normal for twice as many people who took D supplements compared to those who didn't.

Researchers say it's because vitamin D improves inflammation and insulin resistance.

The Recommended Dietary Allowance (RDA) of vitamin D is 600 International Units (IU) if you are younger than 70 years old, and 800 IU if you are over age 70. Those participating in the study took much larger doses — more than 8,500 IU a day for eight weeks, then 2,000 IU a day for the remainder of the study. Talk to your doctor before upping your own vitamin D dose to higher levels.

Let a tiny seed deliver a powerful blow. It's often called a superfood, and no wonder. Flaxseeds contain omega-3 fatty acids, soluble fiber, and plant chemicals called lignans — three champions in the fight against diabetes.

Overweight men and postmenopausal women at high risk for developing diabetes lowered their blood glucose and insulin levels by adding ground flaxseed to their daily diet, shows a *Nutrition Research* study. Just tossing a couple of tablespoons of ground flaxseed on your cereal or yogurt, or into a smoothie, does the trick.

Dim light at night keeps blood sugar just right. It's an hour before bedtime, and if you're like 95 percent of Americans, your eyes are on the TV, your cellphone, a computer, or a video game. It's the age of technology, you say. So what's the big deal?

The big deal is the light from all these devices — called blue-enriched light — has a very short wavelength. You won't notice it, but this light flickers and creates a subtle glare. And that's why your eyes feel tired or you might develop a headache after a day spent working on the computer.

Hold on, though. The news get worse. Exposure to blue light in the evening is linked to cancer, heart disease, obesity, and now, perhaps, diabetes.

> Take a deep breath. That stress you're feeling may put you at higher risk for diabetes. A research team from Rice University in Houston has discovered a link between anxiety and inflammation that may trigger diabetes. They recommend finding ways to manage your stress. See the *Anxiety* chapter for tips.

People in a small study out of Northwestern University, exposed to three hours of blue-enriched light in the evening had higher blood sugar levels than those exposed to dim light. In fact, being around this blue light magnified insulin resistance whether it was during the morning or the evening hours.

"These results provide further evidence that bright light exposure may influence metabolism," says Kathryn Reid, the senior study author and an associate professor at Northwestern.

Some experts think it's the way blue light affects hormones like leptin and melatonin that impacts your body weight, appetite, sleep patterns, and blood sugar levels.

If you simply can't "unplug," at least dim the brightness on your devices. Better yet, try to spend your evenings away from electronics. Create a dimly lit environment, and enjoy a good book or a puzzle.

Why guys need good shut-eye. Men, if you get too much or too little sleep, you could be setting yourself up for diabetes.

A study out of the United Kingdom found that men who slept more or less than the average seven hours were not able to break down sugar properly, even if they were otherwise healthy.

Women, on the other hand, had better glucose levels if they slept longer or shorter than the average, so their diabetes risk did not rise.

Experts think it's because women in general maintain deep sleep for longer, so their blood sugar metabolism remains steady throughout the night. But more men suffer from sleep apnea, which interrupts the deep and restorative sleep stage. This, in turn, results in blood sugar imbalances.

Talk to your doctor if you think you have sleep apnea, then check out these five strategies that will help you get just the right amount of good quality sleep.

▸ Establish a regular bedtime routine.

- Avoid naps.

- Don't exercise too close to bedtime.

- Enjoy an evening bath.

- Keep your bedroom between 60 and 72 degrees Fahrenheit.

Add in an ancient grain — a modern miracle worker.
Holistic doctors in ancient India were on to something when they used barley to treat "sweet urine disease," an early term for diabetes. Maybe they knew they were using the whole grain that's highest in fiber — a whole grain you could easily use today to prevent diabetes.

People who ate bread made primarily with barley kernels at breakfast, lunch, and dinner improved their metabolism, lowered their blood sugar and insulin levels, and felt fuller longer, say Swedish researchers. Scientists give fiber the credit and particularly what fiber does in your gut.

"After eating the bread made out of barley kernel," says Dr. Anne Nilsson, a health science professor at Lund University in Sweden, "we saw an increase in gut hormones that regulate metabolism and appetite, and an increase in a hormone that helps reduce chronic low-grade inflammation among the participants. In time this could help prevent the occurrence of both cardiovascular disease and diabetes."

The bread used in the study combined 85 percent barley kernels with wheat flour. But you can add barley to your meals simply by tossing it into soups, stews, salads, or on the side instead of rice or potatoes. You can even replace your morning oatmeal with barley.

Just make sure you get hulled over pearl barley. Pearl cooks quicker, but hulled retains the nutritious bran and endosperm layer.

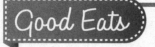

Hunting for 'berried' treasure: a sweet treat to fight diabetes

You have to be quick when shopping for fresh raspberries because they don't last long. Here are some tips to help you enjoy them more.

- Shop for fully ripe raspberries that are aromatic, firm, plump, brightly colored, and have no cores. The core of a ripe raspberry remains attached to the plant, leaving the berry hollow. So, if you find a raspberry with its core intact, that means it was not fully ripe when picked. And raspberries don't ripen after they're harvested.

- Handle raspberries gently. They are very fragile. Wash them quickly in cold water just before using, drain well, and let them air dry, or pat them softly with a paper towel. Don't let them get water-soaked or sit at room temperature too long.

- Freeze raspberries by placing them in a single layer on a cookie tray. After they're frozen, store them in a sealable plastic bag in the freezer.

Give raspberries the red-carpet treatment they deserve. Why cover your salad with fattening croutons when you can sprinkle on red raspberries instead? They're not only delicious, they're chock-full of nutrients that lower diabetes risk. Nutrients like fiber; vitamin C; natural plant chemicals called polyphenols, including anthocyanins and ellagitannins; and a variety of minerals like calcium, magnesium, potassium, and iron. Raspberries are good for you because they:

▶ act as antioxidants against damaging free radicals.

▸ reduce inflammation.

▸ increase insulin levels.

▸ reduce blood sugar levels.

Probiotics protect against insulin resistance. Perhaps you know about the benefits of probiotics and how all those good bacteria keep your digestive tract happy. But did you know probiotics are also potent weapons in your fight against diabetes? Here's how they work.

Remember playing with dominoes — standing them up one behind the other, and then knocking down the first one to watch all the rest fall? That describes what happens in your gut.

First, if you don't have enough good bacteria, your digestive system gets out of balance as the bad bacteria grows. Some experts believe this increases your risk of becoming insulin resistant, possibly by working against chronic inflammation or damage from rogue molecules in your body called free radicals. And with insulin resistance, you're on your way to knocking over that one last domino — the one labeled diabetes.

So how do you keep this domino effect from happening in your body?

Start by eating more vegetables and fewer foods containing animal fat, suggests the Danish research team that studied probiotics' effects on insulin resistance. Then consider getting probiotics from food sources like yogurt, miso soup, and unpasteurized sauerkraut. Taking a probiotic supplement is also a good way to help keep your gut's ecosystem healthy and harmonious, but experts aren't yet ready to recommend a specific strain for controlling blood sugar levels.

2 surprising blood sugar stabilizers

Who Knew?

Creamy whole milk and decadently rich chocolate good for diabetes? No, you're not dreaming.

- Full-fat dairy foods are no longer off limits. The why is still up for debate, but people who drank whole milk weighed less and lowered their chances of getting diabetes when compared to those who drank skim or low-fat. Milk fat contains approximately 400 different fatty acids, and many experts believe these get some of the credit.

- A little bit of chocolate a day — about 3.5 ounces — reduced insulin resistance and improved liver enzymes in more than 1,000 people who were part of the Observation of Cardiovascular Risk in Luxembourg (ORISCAV-LUX) study. Experts believe it's the natural plant chemicals, called polyphenols, in chocolate that make it a nutritional powerhouse. But indulging in this sweet treat comes with a warning. Stick with dark chocolate and continue to exercise, otherwise you could gain weight over time.

The perfect diet? A simple way to slim down

Blood sugar drops. Pounds melt off without trying. Medication remains stable. If you could follow a diet plan that does all that and is super easy to follow, would you do it?

Then say hello to the "structured nutrition plan" developed by diabetes experts in Boston. They have found a way to help overweight and obese people with diabetes, without increasing exercise, changing medications, or adjusting behaviors.

In a nutshell, the structured meal plans looks something like this.

Carbohydrates. Get about 40 percent of your daily calories from carbs, like non-starchy vegetables, minimally processed grains, and fruit.

Fats. These should make up about 30 percent of your daily calories. But not just any fats, only healthy monounsaturated and polyunsaturated fats. The kind you find in nuts, seeds, canola oil, salmon, and tuna.

Protein. No more than 30 percent of your daily calories should come from proteins like fish, lean meat, and legumes.

The plan is also high in fiber, and low in sodium and saturated fats.

"We have been using this structured plan for many years in our Why WAIT (Weight Achievement & Intensive Treatment) program for diabetes weight reduction — with excellent success," says Dr. Hamdy, Medical Director of the Obesity Clinical Program at Joslin Diabetes Center. "Patients frequently ask us for a structured plan and find it easier to follow."

Researchers from the center tested the meal plan on patients with diabetes battling their weight. The group that experienced the most dramatic changes in weight and blood sugar received:

▶ highly structured meal plans based on calories and specific ratios of fats, proteins, and carbohydrates.

▶ menu books.

▶ a snack list.

▶ a supply of calorie replacement foods.

In addition, they were asked to maintain a food log and received phone calls every week from a registered dietitian.

"It was surprising to see all these significant changes in A1C (a measure of blood glucose levels) and body weight without altering medications or activity level and without aiming for weight reduction," says Hamdy, "which tells us that nutrition therapy can be as effective as medications even after a long duration of the disease."

Although the Joslin Diabetes Center's Why WAIT program is only offered in Boston, you can learn more about it online at *www.joslin.org*. Or contact a registered dietitian in your area for guidance.

Mealtime makeover: take time to eat on schedule

What, where, and how you eat are all extremely important factors in staying healthy and maintaining a healthy weight. Now, researchers are focusing on "when."

If you're like most people, you try to go to bed around the same time and get up around the same time. But it's good to have regular mealtimes, too.

They call it "chrono-nutrition" and it's a term used to describe your eating patterns and how they affect your metabolism and your internal body clock. Chrono-nutrition has helped scientists learn that people who have irregular eating patterns — like shift workers — are at higher risk for getting diabetes, cancer, and heart disease.

But even if you're not a shift worker, you could suffer from "social jet lag," which means you skip meals, eat later in the day, and eat out more often. This also increases your risk of diabetes and disease.

Exactly when you pile on the majority of your calories matters, too. "There seems to be some truth in the saying, 'Eat breakfast like a king, lunch like a prince, and dinner like a pauper,' " says Dr. Gerda Pot, visiting lecturer at King's College London. People struggling with their weight, who ate more calories in the morning and fewer in the evening, lost more weight and had better blood sugar levels.

Can this miracle plant manage your diabetes?

New!

Moringa — sounds like something you'd perform on "Dancing With the Stars." But it's actually a tropical plant that boasts the power to heal diabetes, and more.

- Thai researchers found 4,000 milligrams (mg) of moringa powder in capsules boosted insulin production.

- In a separate study, people with diabetes lowered their blood sugar by 21 percent when they took 50,000 mg of moringa powder with a meal.

Because it's jam-packed with nutrients like omega-3 fatty acids, vitamins A and C, iron, protein, calcium, and potassium, moringa battles a whole host of other ailments like ulcers, cancer, bacterial infections, inflammation, and high blood pressure.

Native to Southeast Asia, this "miracle tree," as it is some-times called, also grows in Africa and South America. You can order capsules containing 400 mg of moringa leaf powder from websites like *moringatrees.org*.

Curing the incurable — how you can reverse diabetes

"If a person really wants to get rid of their type 2 diabetes, they can lose weight, keep it off, and return to normal," says Roy Taylor, Professor of Medicine and Metabolism at Newcastle University in England.

Surprised? You're not alone. Experts around the world are learning to think differently about treating this so-called "incurable" disease after a six-month study showed volunteers with long-term diabetes reversed their condition by losing weight.

It was a tough regimen — only 600 to 700 calories a day for eight weeks. Every day the participants had three diet shakes and about a cup of non-starchy vegetables. They could also drink eight cups of calorie-free beverages. Then they began replacing one shake with a meal every three days, gradually returning to a menu of normal food — but eating about a third fewer calories than before the study. In addition, they kept up their level of physical activity throughout.

Participants lost an average of 30 pounds, and six months after they finished the study, had maintained their weight loss and were still diabetes-free.

Researchers think losing weight removes fat from the pancreas, allowing it to return to its normal insulin production.

"This supports our theory of a Personal Fat Threshold," says Taylor. "If a person gains more weight than they personally can tolerate, then diabetes is triggered, but if they then lose that amount of weight, they go back to normal." Just remember, a drastic diet like this one calls for a doctor's supervision.

Is a cure-all pill on the horizon?

New!

A baby aspirin. A statin. A blood pressure pill. A blood sugar tablet. Your pill organizer is busting at the seams.

But what if you could take all those pills and roll them into one convenient capsule? That's what scientists are exploring in a medication they've named the "polypill."

It would include low, relatively safe doses of medications already available with a prescription, like those for heart disease and diabetes, plus a baby aspirin.

You'd need a prescription for this polypill, but who would qualify is still under debate. Some researchers think the polypill would benefit people at high risk for serious diseases. Others think anyone over age 50 should take it as a preventive measure.

The polypill is not currently available for sale in the United States, but you can learn more about one in the United Kingdom by going online at *www.polypill.com*.

Balance the blood sugar beast naturally

Each one of these unusual remedies lowered blood sugar levels in people with diabetes. Just talk to your doctor before adding anything new to your diet.

Vinegar. Two tablespoons of vinegar with lunch and another two with dinner helped people even if they already had their diabetes under control with medication. Experts say it's because vinegar improves insulin production. Don't drink the vinegar straight, however. Add it to your food, perhaps as a balsamic glaze, or mix it with water.

Pistachios. They are chock-full of nutrients like fiber, vitamins, minerals, and healthy unsaturated fats. Perhaps that's why when people with prediabetes ate 2 ounces of pistachios a day, their blood sugar and insulin levels dropped significantly.

Whey protein. A study presented to the Endocrine Society shows people with diabetes who maintained a diet high in whey protein for 12 weeks lost weight and improved their blood sugar levels.

"Whey protein powder, which is a byproduct of milk during cheese production, induced greater satiety and reduction of glucose spikes after meals compared to other protein sources, such as eggs, soy or tuna," explains lead study author Dr. Daniela Jakubowicz, professor of medicine at Tel Aviv University. For a quick breakfast, add it to your shakes and smoothies.

Ginger. Multiple studies found that over a two-month period, taking from 1 to 2 teaspoons of ground ginger a day after meals significantly lowered blood sugar. Scientists think it's all the natural compounds in ginger, especially the gingerols, that keep blood sugar under control.

Grape seed extract. Numerous animal studies suggest grape seed extract could be used to lower blood sugar and manage diabetes. One study out of India even found it boosts the effects of Metformin, a drug used to treat high blood sugar levels caused by type 2 diabetes. Researchers say it's the natural compounds in grapes called proanthocyanidins that promote healthy blood sugar and insulin levels.

Diarrhea

That awful "gotta go" feeling happens to nearly everyone. In fact, diarrhea comes in number two — no kidding — among all reported illnesses in the United States. If you're like most adults, you'll suffer four bouts a year.

Your body's process of elimination. It's supposed to work like this. Let's say you take a big bite of a nice, red apple. The chewed-up bits travel down your esophagus to your stomach, through your small intestine, and into your colon or large intestine. Along the way, the apple pieces get smaller and smaller, and your body pulls out and absorbs all the nutrients it needs — including water. Eventually all that's left of the apple is dry waste material your body expels. The whole process could take anywhere from 12 to 48 hours. Beginning to end, head to tail.

But sometimes food passes too quickly through your digestive system, and your body can't absorb the nutrients and fluids fast enough. The outcome? Loose and watery stools you know as diarrhea.

It hits, you run. Acute diarrhea usually lasts from two days to two weeks. It's often caused by a bacteria, a virus, or even a parasite. It can also be an unpleasant side effect of artificial sweeteners, some medicines, or certain foods. Watch out for diarrhea triggers like fried, fatty, or spicy dishes including Tex-Mex and curries. Some people also have an intense reaction to caffeine, which is known to speed up your digestive system.

Chronic diarrhea lasts longer than acute diarrhea, perhaps more than a month. Some serious disorders like ulcerative colitis, Crohn's disease, irritable bowel syndrome (IBS), and even diabetes are possible causes.

It's time for professional help. Your gut's telling you something's wrong. When should you head to the doctor?

▸ You have a fever of more than 102 degrees.

▸ You become dehydrated. Warning signs include excessive thirst, dry mouth or skin, little or no urination, dizziness, weakness, or dark-colored urine.

▸ Your diarrhea lasts more than two days.

▸ You have severe pain in your abdomen or rectum.

▸ You have black or bloody stools.

If you don't have any of these symptoms, you may be able to treat your condition on your own. Read on for six home remedies sure to get your gut running good as new.

End diarrhea woes with these 6 remedies

Fend off discomfort with a fennel massage. Make a calming rub for your distressed tummy by combining 8 drops of fennel essential oil with 2 tablespoons of your favorite carrier oil. Remember, a carrier or base oil is used to dilute essential oils, making them safer for your skin. Common ones come from vegetables, seeds, or nuts, and include almond, avocado, olive, sesame, sunflower, and jojoba.

Use your fingertips to massage the fennel mixture onto your abdomen. Repeat this treatment three times each day until your diarrhea symptoms subside.

Nothing soothes like a cup of tea. "But indeed I would rather have nothing but tea," said Sir Thomas in Jane Austin's classic "Mansfield Park." And indeed a cup of chamomile tea may just hit the spot when you're experiencing bowel troubles. With its healing properties often compared to China's famous ginseng, chamomile has been used for centuries to relieve diarrhea, nausea, and gas.

Make a delicious, comforting tea by combining 2 or 3 teaspoons of dried chamomile flowers with 1 cup of hot water. Steep covered for 10 to 15 minutes. Or use 1 teaspoon of chamomile root, allowing the tea to steep for 10 to 20 minutes. Strain. Add honey or lemon to taste. Drink 2 to 4 cups daily.

A pinch of allspice will ease your tummy troubles. What do pumpkin pie, pickles, jerky, and ketchup have in common? Recipes for all usually contain the delightful flavor of allspice, a pea-sized berry that tastes and smells like a combination of cinnamon, cloves, ginger, and nutmeg. Besides enjoying it in everything from meatloaf to cookies, you'll want to try allspice for many of your digestive woes, like gas and diarrhea.

To make a soothing tea, add 1 to 2 teaspoons of ground allspice to 1 cup of boiling water. Steep for 15 minutes, and then strain the liquid through a coffee filter. Drink up to 3 cups of allspice tea per day for diarrhea relief.

You can also add a pinch of allspice to a cup of warm milk. If you like, add some sweetness with a little honey. For best results, drink a cup after every bowel movement.

Cinnamon tea gets your gut back on track. The spicy aroma and flavor of cinnamon may make it one of the most beloved condiments in your kitchen. It's versatile enough to pep up a sweet dish or add a subtle warmth to stews and curries. But as popular as it is for cooking, cinnamon has an even longer history in folk medicine. From ancient Egypt and China to Europe in the Middle Ages, herbalists used cinnamon against a slew of digestive ailments. Today, you can whip up your own home remedy in no time.

Start with 4 cups of boiling water. Add 1/4 teaspoon of cayenne pepper and 1/2 teaspoon of cinnamon. Simmer your tea for 5 minutes. Remove from heat and steep for 10 minutes. For flavorful relief from diarrhea, drink 1/4 cup every half hour.

> Cinnamon sticks are perfect for infusing flavor into hot liquids — a job ground cinnamon just can't handle. But don't buy the sticks planning to grind your own. Test kitchens have proven the flavor and texture aren't the same.

Another delicious tea, popular with the Pennsylvania Dutch, combines 1/8 teaspoon of cinnamon, 1 teaspoon of nutmeg, and a little honey in a cup of warm milk. Drink at mealtime to soothe symptoms of diarrhea. For a little extra zing, add a pinch of powdered cloves, like they do in Brazil.

Pick pectin to stop your bellyaching. When diarrhea's got you in its grip, reach for apple cider vinegar. As a natural antiseptic, it cleanses your digestive system. It also contains pectin, a compound found in the cell walls of all plants that adds bulk to your stools and helps put an end to your diarrhea.

Simply add 1 teaspoon of apple cider vinegar to a glass of water. Drink with each meal for some all-natural relief.

Carob — a cure worth its weight in gold. Long ago in ancient Rome, gold and gemstones were weighed against the seeds of the carob tree. Over time, "carob" evolved into "carat." So in ancient terms, if your gold weighed 24 carob seeds, it was said to be 24-carat, or 100 percent pure gold.

But in today's world, it's the pods of the carob plant — not its seeds — that are highly valued. The powdered pods are used in herbal medicines to treat several health conditions, including diarrhea. It works because this carob powder is rich in natural tannins, a substance that dries out the tissues in your digestive tract, reducing inflammation and the amount of fluids your mucous membranes produce.

A daily adult dose of carob powder is 15 to 20 grams, or about 2 to 3 tablespoons. To relieve diarrhea, stir it into a serving of applesauce and enjoy the unique, chocolaty flavor.

A cool treat is just what the doctor ordered

Try this delicious recipe, sure to cure what ails you. In your blender or food processor, combine 1/2 cup almond, rice, or soy milk with 1 frozen banana, 1 teaspoon carob powder, and 1 1/2 teaspoons of honey. Blend until smooth. Enjoy.

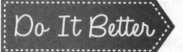

This simple solution keeps you hydrated

Dehydration is a serious concern when you're battling diarrhea — especially for children and seniors. Remember your mother encouraging you to down cups of apple juice, bowls of chicken broth, or bottles of lemon-lime soda? Even a glass of that tangy orange sports drink? Turns out maybe Mom didn't know best. Researchers now say these beverages can actually make your diarrhea worse because they don't have the right balance of nutrients.

Instead, try what's called an oral rehydration salts (ORS) solution to help your body replenish the fluids and nutrients you lose with diarrhea. If you can't run to the store to pick up a commercially produced ORS product like Pedialyte or Hydralyte, you can make your own.

Combine 1/4 teaspoon salt, 1/4 teaspoon baking soda, and 2 tablespoons sugar in 2 cups of water. Sip this solution in small amounts throughout the day to keep your system in balance.

The power of probiotics: 1 great reason to eat yogurt

You probably think of bacteria as germs. And, in many cases, you would be right. But bacteria that live and thrive inside your body are so much more.

Your digestive system, for instance, is home to a staggering 39 trillion, *Science News* reports. And this gut flora, as it is sometimes called, is critical for your digestion to work properly. When you don't have enough good bacteria here you can often feel it, in the form of constipation, gas, diarrhea, or various infections.

So when you suffer from a case of infectious diarrhea, basically your good bacteria are getting trounced by some bad bacteria.

Let probiotics halt your symptoms and save the day. As germ-fighting microorganisms, they are similar to the ones you have naturally in your body, but you get them in capsules, tablets, or powders, and in certain foods, like yogurt, soft cheese, or buttermilk. Take a probiotic and you are literally sending reinforcements straight to your immune system.

One study showed that probiotics can make your infectious diarrhea go away about one day faster. Researchers found two-thirds of those who did not take probiotics were still having diarrhea symptoms after three days. But over half of the people who took probiotics were diarrhea-free in the same amount of time.

Boost good gut bacteria naturally with the right probiotic. How do you decide which strains of bacteria will do the most good? Depends on the cause of your diarrhea.

▶ For diarrhea brought on by a round of antibiotics, look for products that contain *Saccharomyces boulardii*, a strain of baker's yeast, and *Lactobacillus*. For best results, begin taking probiotics as soon as you start taking your medicine, and keep it up for two weeks after you've finished your antibiotics. Be sure to wait at least two hours after you take your antibiotic before you take a probiotic.

▶ Trying to avoid or treat travelers diarrhea? Check labels for products that contain *Saccharomyces boulardii, Lactobacillus acidophilus,* and *Bifidobacterium bifidum.* These three probiotics may be just the ticket for getting — or keeping — your digestive system on a healthy track.

When choosing a probiotic, make sure you're getting enough live cells in every dose. Products can range from 100 million cells to 900 billion per dose. You'll have to do your homework here to determine what you need. And finally, remember there are some situations where taking probiotics is not a healthy decision, so talk to your doctor first.

Dry skin

What do snail mucus, crocodile dung, and sour milk have in common? Why, they're all treatments for dry skin, of course. From long-ago beauty Cleopatra to today's celebrities, the rich and famous have always been on the lookout for better ways to care for their skin.

Snail slime not your style? Don't worry. You can still be red-carpet ready with practical, down-to-earth treatments that give your dry skin a movie-star glow.

Your skin unmasked. Here's the skinny on, well, your skin. As your body's largest organ, its main job is to act as a barrier, protecting your insides from harmful things that lurk outside. It contains countless nerve endings that gauge pain, pressure, and temperature, and send important information back to your brain.

Since you shed dead skin cells day and night — even while you sleep — about every 28 days you get to start fresh with brand-spanking new skin.

> Changes in the way your skin looks can signal changes in your overall health. For example, dry, itchy skin can mean you need a better moisturizer or it could be a warning sign of kidney disease or diabetes. Talk to your doctor if you're concerned.

Face the facts about smart skin care. As you age, the sweat and oil glands that helped naturally moisturize your skin start to dry up, leaving behind those itchy, flaky patches. You can't hold back the hands of time, but there are some steps you can take to hold off dry skin.

▸ Too much heat during the winter and too much air conditioning during the summer can cause bone-dry bodies. A humidifier will help moisten the air — and your skin.

▸ Some antiperspirants and soaps can dry you out, so use them sparingly. Look for products that are marked fragrance-free or hypoallergenic, and avoid those that contain alcohol or dyes.

▸ Certain types of fabric, like wool or synthetic blends, are not skin-friendly. Cotton is your best choice.

Continue reading to find out about a few all-natural remedies, perfect for soothing your parched skin.

Get glowing with these 5 dry skin soothers

A balm to soothe the soul — and your dry skin. Since the Middle Ages, lemon balm has been used to calm anxiety and lower stress levels. Modern herbalists now know this fragrant plant can also be used to ease dry skin. So why not treat your distressed skin to an aromatic steam facial.

Place 1 to 2 tablespoons each of dried lemon balm, chamomile, lavender, and rose petals in a large bowl. Cover the herbs with a quart or two of boiling water. Carefully sit with your face over the bowl, draping a large towel over your head to keep steam from escaping. Inhale the relaxing aromas for several minutes.

Wipe your face with a cool cloth when you're finished, then gently pat your skin dry. To top off your facial, apply moisturizer or toner.

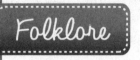

Dousing the water myth: is your skin really thirsty?

A tall, refreshing glass of cool water is the perfect antidote for dry, scaly skin, right? Nope. Experts say there's no evidence that drinking extra H2O has any serious impact on your dry skin.

In fact, other organs in your body are first in line to soak up every drop. Water starts out traveling to your intestines, then through your bloodstream, and then on to your kidneys. Skin cells are close to last on the list.

Of course keeping your body hydrated is important for overall good health. Just don't count on a sip from the tap to fix flaky skin.

Magnesium salt: a mineral miracle for your dry skin. The Dead Sea — which is actually a lake nestled between Jordan, Israel, and the West Bank — is well-known for its healing waters. Rich in minerals, it has a long history of helping those with joint problems, breathing issues, and many chronic skin conditions, including psoriasis.

To test the truth in this tradition, researchers out of Germany had a group of people suffering from atopic dermatitis bathe in the Dead Sea waters every day for six weeks. At the end of the study their skin was significantly smoother, softer, and less inflamed. Experts give credit to the high amount of magnesium chloride in the waters.

Since a trip to the Dead Sea is out of the question for most folks, dermatologists sometimes use a similar, natural treatment of magnesium salt baths for their psoriasis patients.

If you'd like to give this a try at home, talk to your doctor, then look for bags or bottles of magnesium bath flakes. Just remember these two points:

▸ For the most benefit, make sure the product is at least 46 percent magnesium chloride by weight.

▸ And don't mistakenly purchase Epsom salt, which is magnesium sulfate, not magnesium chloride.

Smooth away scaly skin with this floral soak. Both lavender and patchouli oils are known for their skin-soothing properties. Here's a recipe that lets you double down on their benefits.

Combine 3 tablespoons of a carrier oil — like almond, avocado, olive, sunflower, or jojoba oil — with 6 drops each of lavender and patchouli oils in a small bowl.

Simply smooth this over your rough, dry skin or pour the entire mixture into your bath while the warm water is running. Soak for 15 minutes or longer. You can indulge in this fragrant treatment every day, but be very careful getting in and out of the tub. It may be slippery.

A surprising remedy from your fridge. Lactic acid is one of the alpha hydroxy acids (AHAs) you'll find in many moisturizers and exfoliants. AHAs work in two ways. First they scrub away itchy, scaly skin. Then they seal moisture in, leaving your skin feeling oh, so smooth.

You could spend a wad of cash on beauty creams and moisturizers containing AHAs, or you could visit the dairy aisle of your supermarket and pick up fermented milk products like buttermilk, kefir, and yogurt that naturally contain lactic acid.

▸ For a DIY facial, apply plain, full-fat yogurt to your clean face, avoiding the eye area. Leave on for 15 to 30 minutes, then rinse off. Some experts recommend using organic yogurt, while others swear by Greek yogurt. Do a patch test on your skin to see what works best for you.

▸ Dip a cotton ball or a piece of gauze into a bowl of buttermilk, and apply it to your dry, itchy skin for several minutes. Wipe clean with a cloth soaked in tepid water.

▸ Kefir — pronounced kuh-fear' — is a fermented milk drink, rich in beneficial probiotics and nutrients. It has a tangy taste, similar to yogurt, and, like yogurt, contains lactic acid. Make a kefir mask for your dry skin by combining a couple tablespoons of kefir with an egg yolk and a few drops of olive oil. Let this sit on your skin for 10 to 20 minutes. Wash off and gently pat dry.

Olive oil — it's not just for salads anymore. This healthy kitchen staple is chock-full of antioxidants and fatty acids that are not only good for your insides, but they keep your outsides healthy, too.

Try this tip. Before you apply any lotion, dab a little extra virgin olive oil on your skin. It's an easy, inexpensive way to nourish and moisturize.

Or mix up this delightful scrub to oil away dry skin. Start with 1 tablespoon of olive oil. Add 2 tablespoons of fine brown sugar. Stir in 1/2 tablespoon of honey. With your fingertips, rub the mix on your dry skin using circular motions. Scrub lightly for several minutes, and then shower. Apply a light moisturizer to your skin when finished.

Pycnogenol: natural extract says bye-bye dry skin

New!

Could a little-known pine bark extract be the next great thing in skin care? Sure it sounds like something that belongs in a granola recipe, but this natural product, taken from the French maritime pine tree, contains a powerful antioxidant and anti-inflammatory called procyanidin, often used to treat a variety of circulation problems.

So why do you and your dry, lackluster skin care? Because women in a small German study, who took a daily supplement containing procyanidin, found it made their skin smoother, softer, and more hydrated after just 12 weeks.

Experts believe the extract boosts production of hyaluronic acid — a kind of internal lubricant — and collagen — a protein that gives your skin strength and structure.

You can buy pine bark extract as a supplement called Pycnogenol, the brand most widely researched. Even better news, those in the study took just 75 milligrams a day, which will cost you far less than most beauty creams.

Smooth skin secrets every woman should know

The average American woman will spend a whopping $15,000 on cosmetics during her lifetime, reports the personal finance blog Mint.com. And if you have dry skin, tack on an extra bundle for those pricey moisturizers.

Since you're going to invest that kind of money in your makeup, make sure the end result is healthy, glowing skin. Follow these simple tips that are sure to leave your dry skin looking luminous and your makeup flawless.

Moisturize morning and night. Use a thick cream designed especially for dry skin with ingredients to help your skin retain moisture. Apply generously to your face, neck, and chest.

Stay away from powder. Dust a little on your T-zone — forehead, nose, and chin — if you get shiny, but avoid it whenever you can. The same is true of many foundations and other makeup labeled "long-lasting." They can dry out your skin.

Apply your makeup with brushes or sponges only. Touching your face with your fingers can deplete your skin's natural moisture. So for a fresh, dewy look, it's strictly hands off.

Exfoliate once a week. Dead skin can build up on your face, causing your makeup to flake just hours after you apply it. Experts say you should use a gentle exfoliant weekly, and follow up with a good moisturizer. For your lips, use a damp toothbrush — no toothpaste, please — to gently remove dry skin, or scrub away rough patches with a mixture of sugar and honey.

Fight eczema flare-ups with all-natural remedies

Itchy, red, cracked, and leathery. Even some blisters, too. This is more than just run-of-the-mill dry skin. You're battling eczema, a skin condition affecting as many as 30 million Americans.

Maybe you were just born with it. Turns out about 10 percent of infants suffer from some form of eczema. For most, symptoms go away as they get older. But you can also develop one of the seven types of eczema as an adult. It's important to get a proper diagnosis and understand your triggers — which can range from food allergies to chemical irritants, certain fabrics, and even stress.

There's no cure for eczema, but you can relieve its bothersome symptoms in a number of ways.

Renew your skin from the inside out with foods that soothe.
A healthy diet can reduce inflammation, so eat fewer processed foods, cut back on the sugar, and load up on fresh vegetables and whole grains. Then consider these little-known remedies.

▸ How about a cup of tea? Studies suggests that drinking oolong tea may heal the sores common with atopic dermatitis, one form of eczema. Tea contains natural chemicals called polyphenols that work to fight your body's allergic response.

▸ First, make sure eating fish doesn't trigger a flare-up of your symptoms. If you don't show signs of a food allergy, consider adding more fish to your menu. Choose sardines, wild salmon, or tuna to pack in skin-saving omega-3 fatty acids. Not a fish fan? Try a fish oil supplement instead to fight inflammation and ease your eczema symptoms.

Join the team to win out over eczema. One study showed that regular exercise — especially team sports — helped relieve eczema symptoms. And it only took three weeks to see improvements. Researchers say exercise has a positive impact on your emotions and self-esteem. But they caution you should avoid sports when your skin symptoms are at their worst. Otherwise, keep moving.

Phototherapy shines a healing light on your skin. Some skin disorders, like eczema, benefit from a little illumination — especially the ultraviolet light from the sun. Professionals often use special lamps that produce ultraviolet B (UVB) light to help relieve symptoms.

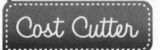

Give dandruff the brush-off with this 2¢ flake fighter

Why pay for dandruff shampoo? Add this bargain-priced ingredient to your regular shampoo, and presto, you've made your own.

Are you among the 50 million Americans trying to head off dandruff? Tired of spending an arm and a leg on expensive treatments? Try this instead.

Crush two uncoated aspirins, and add them to a capful or more of your shampoo. That's all there is to it. The salicylic acid in aspirin helps soften your dry, scaly skin and reduce the scalp inflammation that's causing your dandruff.

When you wash your hair, thoroughly massage the mixture into your scalp. Wait three to five minutes before you rinse. For best results, use every day until you're flake-free.

Falling

The facts are staggering. Did you know one older adult falls every second of every day? And 20 percent of those who suffer a fall are left with broken bones, serious head injuries — or even worse. In 2014, more than 27,000 seniors — 74 every day — died as a result of a fall.

Don't be the fall guy or gal. Here are a few of the common pitfalls you need to avoid.

Your muscles could let you down. Weakness — especially in your legs — is a significant risk factor for falls. Check your strength with the Get Up and Go Test.

To begin, sit in a chair that does not have arms. Without using your arms or hands for support, get up and walk 10 feet. Turn quickly, walk back to the chair, and sit. Have a friend time you. If you take longer than 14 seconds to finish the test, you could be headed toward a tumble.

Infections factor into 45 percent of falls. Urinary and respiratory infections cause confusion, fever, and dizziness — all symptoms that could knock you off your feet. Be on the lookout for early warning signs like weakness or fatigue, and be sure to tell your doctor.

Don't get thrown off balance by low blood pressure. Sometimes blood pressure medications can lower your numbers too much, making you feel dizzy when you stand up. A study of more than 90,000 adults found a 36 percent increase in serious falls during the first two weeks they started taking their medicine.

If you think low blood pressure — or your meds — could be causing problems, ask your doctor to check your orthostatic blood pressure. To do this, he'll compare your blood pressure when you're lying down with your numbers when you stand up. If there's something wrong, he'll figure out the right prescription to keep you steady on your feet.

Get your vision and hearing up to speed. Are all five of your senses up to snuff? If not, you could be asking for trouble. Here are just a couple of examples why.

▶ Cataracts, glaucoma, and problems with depth perception can lead to falls. Even wearing multi-focal lenses — like bifocals — can cause you to stumble. Be sure your eyeglasses fit properly, and get your eyes examined regularly.

▶ A recent study found that people with even a mild hearing loss were nearly three times more likely to have a fall. Researchers think people who can't hear well may not be aware of everything that's going on in their environment, making them more prone to falling. Talk to your doctor about scheduling a hearing test. Just one more way to stay strong and steady.

Now that you know some of the reasons you might stumble, learn how you can get a better grip on slips.

3 ways to avoid slips, trips, and falls

Live a stronger, balanced life. When you hear the term "strength training," what image comes to mind? A muscle-bound he-man lugging around heavy dumbbells? Well, it's time to rethink the stereotype.

Today, experts recommend strength training for anyone who wants to stay steady on their feet and overcome a fear of falling. This type of exercise — also called resistance or weight training — builds up your core. Those are your abdominal and back muscles that help you swing a tennis racquet, push a vacuum, and everything in between. Make them stronger and you can restore your balance at any age, allowing you to live an active, independent life.

Check out books or watch videos to learn the basic moves, or head to your local gym or senior center for help. Then start slowly with a simple 20-minute routine two or three times per week, using free weights or resistance bands. If they're not available, just grab a couple of items from around the house — like soup cans or water bottles. And remember to talk to your doctor before you begin any new exercise routine.

Stay steady on your feet. How are your gait and balance? Can you stand on one leg for 30 seconds without using your hands to brace yourself? Can you walk heel-to-toe, one foot directly in front of the other, without toppling over? Flunking either test could mean a fall is in your future. But practicing these simple balance exercises might get you a passing grade — and keep you fall-free.

 ▶ **One-legged stand.** Position yourself behind a sturdy chair. Raise one foot off the floor and hold for 10 seconds. You can hang on to the chair for support if you need to. Repeat this exercise 10 times with one leg, and then switch to the other leg. Make it more difficult by gripping the chair with just one hand, or by letting go completely. Try it with your eyes closed for an extra challenge.

▶ **Tightrope walk.** Raise your arms to each side, about shoulder-high. Focus on a spot in front of you to help keep you steady. Walk in a straight line, putting one foot in front of the other. As you walk, lift your back leg and hold for one second before moving ahead. Take 20 steps, lifting and holding alternate legs.

▶ **Toothbrush balance.** While standing at the sink brushing your teeth, slightly lift your right foot. Use your right hand to brush the upper left corner of your mouth for 30 seconds — or about the amount of time it takes to hum the "Happy Birthday" song twice. Next, hold the toothbrush in your left hand, raise your left foot, and brush the upper right corner of your mouth for 30 seconds. For extra practice, repeat the exercise on both sides.

Smooth moves keep you stable. Ease into exercise with tai chi, Harvard Medical School's top pick for improving your balance and lowering your risk of falls.

This ancient Chinese art teaches you gentle, flowing movements, performed while you slowly shift your weight and stretch. Because tai chi puts minimal stress on your muscles and joints, it's an exercise program that's generally safe for all ages and all fitness levels. You can do tai chi anywhere — indoors or out — and there's no special equipment required. Do it alone, or sign up for a class.

And it's not just for better balance. Tai chi offers these other health benefits, too.

▶ better mood and less anxiety

▶ improved flexibility and agility

▸ lower blood pressure

▸ reduced inflammation

▸ increased energy

Take a peek at tai chi. Observe a class to see if it's right for you. Check with your local senior center or community education center for a class schedule. Also, the Arthritis Foundation has created a 12-movement, easy-to-learn tai chi routine that might be just what you need. Go online to *resourcefinder.arthritis.org* and search under Fitness Programs to see if there's a class near you.

Try it out at home. You'll find lots of DVDs to teach you the basic moves. And Georgia's Piedmont Hospital system even offers a complete tai chi class you can access online. Go to *piedmont.org* and type "tai chi class" in the search box.

If you have health issues like joint problems, back pain, or severe osteoporosis, be sure to talk to your doctor before trying tai chi. He may want you to avoid or modify some of the postures.

Fix dizziness with a twist

You're standing still, but the room is spinning. Your ears are ringing. You feel nauseated. Your eyes are making strange, jerking movements, and you feel like you're going to fall at any minute.

This is more than just simple dizziness. You're suffering from vertigo. And you're not alone. Nearly 40 percent of adults have had the same experience. Want to know how to conquer it with a simple treatment you can do at home? Just imagine. No doctors. No fees.

Your vertigo is probably caused by a condition called benign paroxysmal positional vertigo, or BPPV. When you have BPPV, tiny calcium deposits called canaliths break free and float around inside your ear canal. These canaliths muddle the messages your inner ear is trying to transmit to your brain about balance, sending you into a tailspin.

The Epley maneuver can put an end to vertigo by moving the canaliths out of your ear canals. Just follow these simple steps.

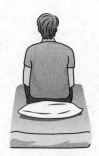

1. Start by sitting upright on your bed. Position a pillow behind you so that when you lie back, it will be under your shoulders, and your head will rest on the bed.

2. Tilt your head back slightly and turn it about 45 degrees to the side of your affected ear. Lie back quickly.

3. After 30 seconds, turn your head 90 degrees to the other side. Keep your head tilted back slightly.

4. Wait 30 seconds. Then turn your whole body 90 degrees so that you are lying on your side. Keep your head in line with your body.

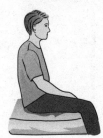

5. After another 30 seconds, push up to a sitting position. Your legs should be hanging over the side of your bed.

That's it. Don't bend over for the rest of the day — it's important you keep your head in an upright position. And for several days after treatment, avoid sleeping on the side that triggers your symptoms.

The Epley maneuver usually works very quickly. However, you can repeat it three times a day until you are vertigo-free for 24 hours.

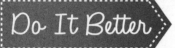

Tricks of the tread: stay safe on your treadmill

When the weather takes a turn for the worse, keep your workout on track by walking on a treadmill. Just be sure to tread safely by following these tips.

- Always use the treadmill's safety key. One end plugs into your machine, and the other clips onto your clothing. If you slip, the key pops out of the treadmill, causing the belt to stop.

- Begin your workout by standing on either side of the belt. Hold onto the handrails as you start the treadmill at a low speed. Carefully step onto the belt, increasing its speed as you adjust your pace.

- Keep your head up and your eyes focused forward. If you look down, you could lose your balance and fall.

- Don't hold onto the handrails. You'll get the best workout — and improve your balance — if you walk at a normal pace and allow your arms to move naturally by your side.

Foot pain

Over the course of a normal day, you pound your heels down on the floor over 8,000 times. And each step you take puts pressure on your feet that's equal to at least three times your own body weight. Running and other active sports just add to that jarring and stress. Is it any wonder your feet are prone to painful problems?

Foot pain stems from a variety of reasons — ingrown toenails, corns, fallen arches, and strains, just to name a few. So how do you know what's causing your foot pain?

Watch for signs of aging. As you get older, your feet slowly change their shape and size. So watch out for signs of age-related foot pain.

▸ Hammertoes, or claw toes, are caused by tightening ligaments in your foot. Your toes curl downward, taking the shape of a claw. Most shoes will painfully press against the tops of your toes, so look for a wide pair with square, boxy toes.

▸ Bunions are bony growths that form at the joint where your toe meets your foot. They're caused by shoes constantly pushing your toes together. To prevent bunions, wear soft, wide shoes or sandals with plenty of wiggle room.

▸ Fat pads on the bottoms of your feet act like a car's shock absorbers. But as you get older, they began to wear thin, so make sure you wear sturdier, cushioned shoes.

Heel pain points to plantar fascitiis. If your heels are howling before you take your first steps in the morning, you could have plantar fasciitis. It occurs when the ligament that connects your heel bone to your toes becomes swollen and inflamed. You might be at particularly high risk for this problem if you:

▸ frequently walk on unstable surfaces like sand.

▸ have flat feet or high arches.

▸ are overweight.

▸ have a job that involves a lot of walking and standing on hard surfaces.

> If your foot pain is severe or accompanied by tingling, numbness, leg cramps, or fever, see your doctor.

▸ have tight calf muscles that limit the flexibility of your ankles.

▸ have problems with your walking gait.

Treat plantar fasciitis — and other sources of foot pain — with rest, anti-inflammatories like aspirin or ibuprofen, and the following easy tips.

Walk away from foot pain with 3 simple steps

Stretch to soothe your soles. There's no better way to relieve your foot pain than to keep your muscles strong and relaxed. Do these stretches every day to fight off aches and prevent new injuries.

▸ Place a golf ball or a can of frozen fruit juice concentrate on the floor and gently roll your foot over it with light pressure. This gives you the added benefit of an ice massage.

▶ Stand facing a wall. Place your heel on the floor and your toes up on the wall. Push against the wall to gently stretch your heel and the bottom of your foot.

▶ Sit on the floor with your painful foot stretched out in front of you. Wrap a towel around the bottom of your foot, and hold the two ends of the towel in your hands. Gently pull back on the towel to stretch your foot.

▶ Stand with only the front half of both feet on a step. Hold on to something for balance and gently sink your heels down toward the floor.

Kick your old shoes to the curb. Three out of every four people suffering from heel pain are women. And it's usually because of their shoe closet. Don't sacrifice your health for style. Instead, use these tips to tame the pain.

▶ Ditch the heels. They force your feet into an unnatural position and cause tendon and joint damage. If you must wear heels, stick with ones 2 inches high or less. And by the way, completely flat shoes with thin soles and no support can be just as bad for your feet as heels.

▶ Your shoes aren't like fine wine — they don't get better with age. While they may seem comfortable, you should replace worn-out shoes and get ones that fit well and have good support.

Ingrown toenails are painful, but easy to avoid. When you're clipping your nails, trim them straight across the top, not rounded at the edges. Keep your nails long enough so the edges don't get embedded in the skin. You can also wear sandals or open-toed shoes to put less pressure on your toenails.

▶ If you haven't had your feet measured in a while, do it now. Your feet get longer and flatter as you age, so your current shoes could be two sizes too small.

Insert some pep in your step. Finding fashionable shoes with great arch support and enough toe room is nearly impossible. Even when you're lucky enough to find a pair that works, they still feel like they're missing something. Fortunately, you can slip orthotic inserts into your shoes and make every pair fit like Cinderella's slippers.

For most foot pain, you can get relief with over-the-counter inserts like a soft silicon heel cushion or a bunion shield pad. They are available at most drugstores.

However, if you have a serious problem, splash out some cash for custom inserts. They can cost hundreds of dollars and require a doctor's exam, but if you have very flat feet or one leg that's shorter than the other, they're worth it. Insurance may even cover the cost.

When choosing an orthotic, make sure it's designed to help your problem. Wearing the wrong insert will just make your pain worse, so here's a quick guide to choosing the right one.

Foot problem	Recommended item
bunions	bunion shield pad
flat feet	semi-rigid insert, long arch pad, inner heel wedge, or extended heel counter
hammer toe	toe crest pad
plantar fasciitis	prefabricated heel insert

Forgetfulness

Ever wonder where you left your keys? Or why you walked into a room? Or your favorite hairdresser's name — you know, the one you've been to a dozen times over the past couple of years? You're not alone.

"Senior moments" are a normal part of life. Experts say you have them because your brain physically changes as you age. Certain areas shrink and your memory processing speed slows down. But that doesn't mean your occasional lapses are necessarily serious, like dementia or Alzheimer's disease.

Reasons you feel like you've become a bit more forgetful lately could include the following.

Medications. Seems like the older you get, the more you take. And some of them, like sleeping pills, anti-anxiety medications, painkillers, antihistamines, and antidepressants, could trigger memory lapses. Talk to your doctor if you think a new drug is messing with your mind.

Stress. Feeling anxious can wreak havoc on your brain. A 20-year University of Pittsburgh study found that chronic life stress led to a decrease in the volume of the hippocampus, a brain region essential for learning and memory. Other studies have linked high levels of stress hormones to worse memory, focus, and problem-solving skills. That makes sense, because a barrage of stress hormones can shrink brain cells and disrupt connections between them.

Depression. It goes both ways. Feeling down can make you forgetful. And forgetfulness can make you feel down. See your doctor if you can't seem to shake the blues.

Fatigue. Lack of sleep can make you feel seriously pooped out and unable to recall what someone said to you five minutes ago.

Alcohol. Not only does booze lower your ability to remember, your forgetfulness can last after the effects of alcohol have worn off. If you drink at all, stick with no more than two drinks a day for guys and one for gals.

Medical conditions. An underactive thyroid, kidney problems, or liver disorder can mess with your memory. Ask your doctor to test for these serious health issues.

While forgetfulness can be frustrating, there's plenty you can do to fight it. Check out these ways to train your brain to remember.

7 ways to boost your memory

Sweet slumber keeps memories from slipping away. Want to keep your memory sharp as a tack? Then say hello to a good night of shut-eye. Sleep not only boosts your ability to remember, it's the secret to staying mentally alert as you age.

British researchers asked two groups of people to learn a list of made-up words. They tested recall in both groups immediately following the exercise. They then tested one group after a 12-hour period of being awake, and the other after a night of sleep. The group that got sleep was better able to remember the words.

"Sleep almost doubles our chances of remembering previously unrecalled material," says Dr. Nicolas Dumay of the University of Exeter in England. "The post-sleep boost in memory accessibility may indicate that some memories are sharpened overnight."

The part of your brain called the hippocampus helps you recollect newly learned material and experiences by replaying memories to an area of the brain that first captured them. So in essence, your brain relives that day's major events while you sleep and then locks in those memories.

Bet on beta carotene to boost your brain power. Take a bite of a carrot stick or a forkful of sweet potatoes and what do you get? A heaping helping of beta carotene, that's what. This natural plant chemical, which your body converts to vitamin A, acts as a powerful antioxidant to boost brain function and brain cell survival as well as improve communication between brain cells.

▶ The Physicians' Health Study II, which followed nearly 6,000 men age 65 or older, found that those who took beta carotene supplements for 15 years or longer scored slightly higher on memory tests than those who took supplements for three years or less.

▶ And a seven-year study out of the University of California, Los Angeles, determined that high blood levels of beta carotene may protect against mental decline in older people who carry a certain gene that makes them more susceptible to Alzheimer's disease (AD).

That may all sound fine and dandy, but taking beta carotene supplements doesn't come without warnings. For instance, smokers are at higher risk of lung cancer if they take supplements.

Of course, supplements aren't the only way to get beta carotene. Carrots and sweet potatoes are two rich sources. Or if you're feeling more exotic, pick up a mango — it's the tropical fruit that will help you think more clearly as you age.

Charge up your memory with 2 of your favorite things

Who Knew?

Sleep and chocolate team up to fight forgetfulness? How fabulous is that?

New research says after learning something new, a reward — can you say chocolate? — helps lock in the memory. "Rewards may act as a kind of tag, sealing information in the brain during learning," says researcher Dr. Kinga Igloi of the University of Geneva.

Chocolate is a great choice because it contains natural compounds, like flavanoids, caffeine, and theobromine, that promote alertness and guard against mental decline.

Then taking even a short snooze further reinforces the memory. During sleep, the information gets moved to areas of the brain associated with long-term memory. "We already knew that sleep helps strengthens memories," says Igloi, "but we now also know that it helps us select and retain those that have a rewarding value."

So the next time you need to really absorb new info, remember to eat a piece of chocolate and take a nap.

Herbs keep your memory sharp. An old Chinese proverb says, "There are no worthless herbs — only the lack of knowledge."

Consider yourself informed, because what you're about to read is all about five herbs you won't want to forget. Here's the list.

▸ **Peppermint.** Drinking this delightfully aromatic tea not only makes you feel chipper, it helps your working and long-term memory, found a British study. So if you want to keep your mind razor-sharp throughout the day, enjoy a spot of peppermint tea at 9 in the morning, 2 in the afternoon, and 7 at night.

▸ **Sage.** Take sage oil supplements or a whiff of this perennial herb and you'll boost your mood and your memory. Scientists think sage works not only as a powerful antioxidant but also by triggering the release of acetylcholine, a natural brain chemical used by nerve cells to send signals to other cells.

▸ **Cinnamon.** This super versatile spice improved the working memory of people over age 60 with prediabetes, shows a study published in the journal *Nutrition Research*. Ground cinnamon also prompted mice who were "poor learners" to have better recall by actually boosting levels of brain chemicals responsible for memories and decreasing other chemicals that interfere with brain function.

▸ **Rosemary.** Filling your house with the sweet fragrance of rosemary oil could help you recall past events and help you remember to carry out future plans. That's what a small study out of the United Kingdom discovered. Experts believe a compound that gives rosemary its scent triggers a brain chemical responsible for memory.

▸ **Clove.** Herbalists believe cloves contain the power to battle memory loss as well as a host of other ailments like depression, anxiety, and insomnia. Try adding cloves to your tea or to your favorite soups and stews. Or simply enjoy the fragrance.

Warning

The fat that's killing your brain

Trans fatty acids may increase the shelf life of foods, but they will cut your brain's life short if you're not careful.

Created when food manufacturers add hydrogen to vegetable oil, a process known as hydrogenation, trans fats are also called partially hydrogenated oils. They are added to baked goods, margarine, shortening, and fried foods to make the flavor last longer.

"Trans fat consumption has previously shown adverse associations to behavior and mood — other pillars of brain function," says Dr. Beatrice Golomb, professor of medicine at the University of California. "However, to our knowledge a relation to memory or cognition had not been shown."

Not until her research team conducted their study, that is. They discovered that men who ate higher amounts of food with trans fats scored lower on memory tests. So if you've been thinking about giving up cupcakes, cookies, biscuits and frozen pizzas for your waistline, start today for the sake of your brain, too.

Beef up your B12 to benefit your brain. Sharpen your memory — with steak? It sounds too amazing to be true, but it is. That's because steak is loaded with B12, a vitamin long-revered for its ability to keep your mind sharp and your memories intact. Here's how it works.

When you have low levels of B12 and other B vitamins, you typically have high levels of an amino acid called homocysteine. And that increases your risk of mental decline and memory loss. In fact, it even means a greater threat of dementia and Alzheimer's disease.

Some scientists believe that getting more B12 in your diet lowers homocysteine, thereby fending off memory problems.

You get B12 primarily from animal products like meat, fish, eggs, poultry, and dairy, or from fortified grains like cereals. Unfortunately, as you get older your stomach doesn't produce enough acid to absorb B12. Other factors can also contribute to low B12 levels, like a poor diet, too much alcohol, and certain medications.

Have your doctor check you for vitamin deficiencies before increasing B12 on your own.

Bring back old memories by learning new skills. At age 65, Linda took up painting, French, and chess. That's exactly what she needed to do to keep her mind sharp. But now research from a University of Texas study suggests trying new, mentally challenging activities like these could keep her memories alive and well, too.

Older adults who learned quilting, digital photography, or both, and engaged in these activities for around 16 hours a week for three months, were better able to recall "episodic" memories when compared to seniors who spent the same amount of time on activities where they did not have to learn anything new.

These episodic memories are your recollections of experiences and specific events — rather like a newsreel of your life, complete with emotions and sensations. Experts think they improve more than other mental skills because they rely heavily on existing knowledge and your brain's organizational strategies.

Scientists noted that the photography classes were the most demanding because participants also had to learn new computer skills and photo-editing software. Quilting, on the other hand, was more repetitive once participants learned the initial skill.

What's good for your body is good for your brain. Working out keeps your body healthy. But did you know it can keep your brain healthy, too?

▸ Seventy-two people completed a memory activity, then were divided into three groups. One group worked out immediately. One group waited four hours, then worked out. And the final group did not exercise. Two days later all were tested to see how much they remembered.

Surprisingly, those who waited and then exercised had the highest recall scores. And those who exercised immediately had the lowest. Experts from the Netherlands study say exercise changes the way your brain stores memories, perhaps because physical activity releases certain brain chemicals. But delaying that exercise a bit could give those memories time to solidify.

▸ Looks like pumping a little iron may help aging brains, too. Women between 65 and 75, who did light upper- and lower-body weight training, had better brain scans than women who either weight trained once a week or who performed balance and flexibility exercise. Prior to the study, scans showed lesions in all the women's brains — lesions known to affect memory and thinking. And while the lesions grew and multiplied in everyone, the women who did light resistance training twice a week had the least progression.

▸ A small study out of England found people who were over-weight or obese scored poorly on memory tests. Experts think it's because excess weight physically changes your brain and how it works. Hard hit are the specific areas asso-ciated with memory.

Your brain's need for speed improves your memory. Ever feel like your mind is working slower than molasses? As you age, your ability to process informa-tion shifts into a lower gear, and this interferes with your recollection of experiences. But experts say you can train your brain to think quickly and improve your memory.

Apparently, sex makes for a sharper mind. Sexually active men and women over age 50 scored higher on tests of memory skills than those who abstained, shows a British study. Experts aren't sure why, but it's one more good reason to stay "busy" as you age.

▸ **Listen to classical music.** See if you can make out individual instruments like the flute, cello, or snare drum. Honing the skill to separate sounds improves your ability to process new information. Plus, listening to classical music boosted learning and memory on a genetic level, found a Finnish study.

▸ **Play board games.** Research out of France shows people who played board games were 15 percent less likely to get dementia than non-players. Try chess and checkers for strategy, Password and Taboo to build listening skills, and Chinese checkers for logic.

▸ **Participate in sports.** Think quickly, act fast — that's the name of the game when you engage in activities like pickleball or tennis. And all that action pushes your brain to process rapidly.

▸ **Play video games.** Next time your kids and grandkids come over, turn on the Wii or have a couple of games, like Space Fortress, handy on your tablet. Studies show these improve memory skills, mental processing speed, ability to change tasks, and decision-making.

Practical tips to remember the little things

If you've got a frustrating case of absentmindedness, take heart. Even though the ability to remember can become more challenging as you get older, these easy tips will help jog your memory.

Start your day with coffee. Middle-aged people who drank three to five cups every day were 65 percent less likely to develop Alzheimer's disease or other dementias in their later years than those who drank little or no coffee.

Turn off technology. The more time you spend "plugged in," the more forgetful you are — even when you're not connected. A British study found heavy cellphone and internet users struggled with daily life activities, like remembering appointments and simply paying attention.

Focus on one thing. Multitasking can lead to distractions. Instead, think about what you want to learn and remember, and limit the amount of information you take in at one time. Focus on that and nothing else.

Close your eyes. When you're wracking your brain trying to remember something, shut your peepers. Your brain will block other distractions and help you recall more exactly.

Organize information into categories. For instance, if you're taking a trip, group your mental packing list by type of item — shirts, pants, accessories, and toiletries.

Turn off the tunes. Research shows background music could be enough of a distraction to keep you from committing things to memory. Experts suggest you ditch the music when you're learning something new.

Use your eyes, ears, and imagination. Write down what you need to remember, say it out loud, then picture it. If you want to remember someone's name, for example, jot it down and say it repeatedly as you visualize what he or she looks like.

Eat, drink, and beat Alzheimer's disease

One day Joseph asked Barbara, his wife of 40-plus years, to fetch a couple of sodas from the basement refrigerator. She came back with three eggs. A few days later she placed chicken breasts on the kitchen counter to defrost. They sat there all day. She couldn't remember why she took them out. This was not normal, age-related forgetfulness. This was Alzheimer's disease (AD).

As you get older, you may start to wonder if your absentmindedness is the beginning of this dreadful condition. But there's a big difference between everyday brain cramps and full-blown AD. See some examples on the next page.

Don't sweat it	Seek help
You misplace your keys.	You find your keys, but don't know what to do with them.
You forget to pay a monthly bill.	You don't remember how to pay your bills.
You can't find something, but you can retrace your steps.	You can't find something and accuse others of stealing it.
Occasionally you can't recall a word.	You stop in the middle of a sentence and don't know how to continue the conversation.
You forget what day it is, but can figure it out on your own.	You've lost track of the day, the month, and the season.
You accidentally leave out an ingredient in a recipe.	You have trouble following a recipe you've made dozens of times.
You need a minute to remember how to get somewhere.	You don't know where you are.
You don't remember the name of someone you just met.	You don't remember the names of your children and grandchildren.
You give up a favorite hobby because you physically can't do it anymore.	You give up a favorite hobby because you don't remember how to do it anymore.

Still worried? Don't be. Adding healthy fruits and vegetables to your daily menu is one of the best things you can do to prevent Alzheimer's disease. Experts say it's the natural antioxidants called polyphenols in produce that protect your brain, boost your memory, and help fight the disease. In fact, people who drank fruit and vegetable juices at least three times a week were 76 percent less likely to develop Alzheimer's than people who drank it less than once a week.

You can get this powerful nutrient from delicious foods like blueberries, strawberries, blackberries, plums, and spinach.

Clear the haze with this de-lish glaze

Here's a recipe for a yogurt-curry glaze that delivers a one-two punch in the battle against dementia. How? The vitamin D and curcumin found in these foods work together to keep your brain healthy.

- Scientists say vitamin D slows the production of beta-amyloid, a protein that clumps together in your brain to form dangerous plaques linked to Alzheimer's.

- Curry powder contains the spice turmeric. And turmeric gets its yellow color from a compound called curcumin, which works alongside vitamin D to stimulate your immune system and clear the excess beta-amyloid out of your brain.

To make this yummy glaze for grilled salmon, whisk 3/4 cup plain, vitamin D-fortified yogurt with 2 teaspoons minced garlic. Add 1 1/2 teaspoons curry powder, 1/2 teaspoon ground ginger, 2 teaspoons fresh minced cilantro, 1/2 teaspoon lemon zest, and 1/2 teaspoon sugar. Salt and pepper to taste.

Gum disease

Stroke. Bone loss. Breast cancer. Alzheimer's disease. Pancreatic cancer. They all have one surprising thing in common — gum disease. Let oral health slide, and you put yourself at higher risk for all of these terrifying conditions.

It starts when plaque, a sticky film of bacteria, forms along and under your gum line. Germs overrun your mouth, and your immune system gets the message to attack. That may sound like a good thing, but the skirmish actually damages your gum tissue and causes swelling.

"Just like your skin is your first line of defense against illness for your body, so are your gums," says Elise Robinson, a registered dental hygienist in Atlanta. "If your gums are compromised by inflammation, bacteria can spread quickly throughout your body."

That bacteria could trigger cancer and other illnesses. For now, experts only recognize there's a link between certain health problems and sick gums, with inflammation playing a major role.

There are two types of gum disease.

Gingivitis. This mild form causes red, swollen, and bleeding gums. Sounds painful. But it's often not. In fact, many people don't

Keep your dentures clean and germ-free to protect your gums. Scrub them daily with a soft toothbrush and denture cleaner, rinse thoroughly, and soak them overnight in a water-based solution. You'll be ready to show off your toothy grin every morning.

know they have gingivitis because it causes little to no discomfort. A combination of good oral care at home plus treatment at the hands of your dentist can easily reverse gingivitis.

Periodontitis. Leave gingivitis untreated, and things go from bad to worse — you end up with periodontitis. Your gums pull away from your teeth forming spaces or pockets where bacteria thrive. The soft tissue and bone that support your teeth become damaged. Your teeth loosen and may have to be removed. Professional help is your only solution.

Your best course of action is to stop gum disease before it ever takes root. You have the power to do so by following steps that have been drilled into your head for years.

▶ Brush and floss daily.

▶ Visit your dentist regularly.

▶ Eat a healthy diet including foods that lower inflammation — nuts, fruit, legumes, vegetables, and fatty fish, like salmon.

▶ Drink plenty of fluoridated water. Experts say it's the No. 1 beverage for healthy teeth.

Here are a few extra things you can do — things guaranteed to put a smile on your face for years to come.

5 tips to guard your gums against disease

Chew on this: minty gum is your mouth's new best friend. Wipe out 100 million germs in 10 minutes. That's what a simple stick of gum can do in your mouth.

The bacteria actually end up on the chewed piece of gum. And the longer you chew, the more it collects.

Now don't go running to the store for a big bag of pink bubblegum. It may be fun to chew, but all that sugar will just feed the bacteria in your mouth. Stick with sugar-free gum. Artificial sweeteners, like xylitol, not only battle plaque buildup on your teeth, but also kill bacteria that get trapped in the chewing gum. What's more, spearmint and peppermint flavors are antimicrobial, which simply means they can fight off bacteria and stop them from growing.

Bug buddies — let probiotics save your smile. One creamy treat you already love can help keep your teeth and gums strong and give you the confidence boost that comes with a clean, healthy mouth.

Along with tooth-strengthening calcium and protein, yogurt contains millions of "good" bacteria, called probiotics. These are found naturally in your body as well as in foods and supplements. These beneficial microbes help your body by curbing the growth of harmful bacteria, encouraging good digestion, boosting your immune system, and bumping up your resistance to infection.

> Look for chewable tablets or lozenges containing the probiotic *Lactobacillus reuteri*. It has improved chronic gum disease in clinical trials.

What a lot of people don't know is that these good guys are also amazingly helpful in your mouth.

In one study, people took tablets containing probiotic bacteria three times a day. After just eight weeks, scientists saw less plaque buildup and inflammation in gum tissue compared to those who didn't take probiotics.

Like probiotics, lactic acid is made in your body and also found in foods like yogurt. Researchers discovered that foods rich in lactic acid help protect against infection in the spaces between gums and teeth, as well as tissue damage, both telltale signs of gum disease.

Avoid common buying mistakes by following these tips to ensure you get the most out of your yogurt.

▶ Check the sugar content, and beware of fake fruit. You don't want to undo all the good things about yogurt by eating products jam-packed with sugar and artificial ingredients.

▶ Look for "Live and Active Cultures" on the label to insure it contains significant amounts of probiotics. If you don't see this seal, check the ingredient list for *L. bulgaricus*, *S. thermophilus*, or *L. acidophilus*.

A delightful drink suits your teeth to a "T." Move over mouthwash — you've been replaced by green tea, a tastier alternative with powerful plaque-fighting compounds.

That's what a research team out of India discovered. They asked a group of 110 men to rinse their mouths for one minute, twice a day. Half used a mouthwash with 2 percent green tea. The other half rinsed with a placebo mouthwash. After 28 days, the guys that swished green tea had healthier gums and less plaque buildup than the others.

Are you more of a tea-sipper than a tea-swisher? Then go ahead and fill up your cup. People who drank green tea regularly had healthier gums than those who drank less, reports a study published in the *Journal of Periodontology*. In fact, for every extra daily cup the men in the study sipped, their indicators of gum disease went down.

Experts believe natural chemicals in green tea leaves, called catechins, act as an antioxidant to fight inflammation.

So when it comes to your oral health, a little green tea every day may be worth all the tea in China.

> **Warning**
>
> ## Slim down to preserve your pearly whites
>
> Need another reason to lose weight? Look in the mirror, and smile. Those extra pounds could mean a higher risk of gum disease.
>
> When you are overweight, your body reacts with a constant low level of inflammation. And some experts believe this is the link to periodontitis.
>
> Add in unhealthy habits that contribute to weight gain — like smoking, drinking alcohol, eating bad fats and carbohydrates — and your risk climbs even higher.

One "E"ssential way to keep inflammation at bay. Load up your shopping cart with nuts, whole grains, and leafy greens, and you've just armed yourself with foods rich in vitamin E — an antioxidant that works as an anti-inflammatory to shrink your risk of gum disease.

People with low levels of vitamin E had higher rates of gum disease, shows a study published in *The Journal of Nutrition*. In fact, those

with the least amount of vitamin E in their blood were 65
percent more likely to have
gum disease than those with
the highest levels.

Other antioxidants should be
on your radar as well. Fruits
and vegetables, especially those
rich in beta carotene and vitamin C, helped people with
gum disease heal after a deep
cleaning procedure to remove
plaque. Choose brightly colored produce like cantaloupe
and mango, sweet peppers
and broccoli.

> People with periodontitis
> who took a daily combo
> of 81 milligrams (mg) of
> aspirin and 2,000 mg of
> docosahexaenoic acid
> (DHA) in capsules
> reduced the amount of
> inflammation around their
> gums. DHA is an omega-3
> fatty acid found in fatty
> fish. Scientists think
> aspirin causes the DHA to
> change in such a way that
> it helps produce anti-
> inflammatory compounds.

Go natural — make your own healing mouthwash. When
organic forces face off against gum disease, something miraculous
happens — your mouth heals. That's what researchers discovered
when they put these remedies to the test.

▶ **Aloe vera.** It's not just for sunburns anymore. Multiple
studies show you can use the gel to treat periodontitis,
especially if you apply it directly to your gums. While
researchers have injected it into infected pockets, you can
try massaging it in, then rinsing. Make your own aloe
mouthwash with pure gel and water, or look for aloe-based
dental products online or at your local health food store.

Dentist and researcher Dr. Dilip George suggests you check
out nonprofit associations such as the International Aloe

Science Council to see what products have received the organization's seal of quality. You'll find them online at *iasc.org*.

▸ **Herbal rinses.** If you really want to go all-natural, reach for
sage, calendula, or geranium. Herbalists say these three
heavenly herbs heal infected and inflamed gums due to
their antibacterial and anti-inflammatory properties. Make
a mouthwash by steeping dried leaves or mixing an ounce
of tincture with several ounces of distilled water.

Rx Alert

Dry mouth from drugs?
It's riskier than you think

Ever feel like you've swallowed a mouthful of cotton balls?
Then you may have dry mouth syndrome, a condition you
might blame on simply getting older. But there are some
surprising causes of dry mouth that have nothing to do
with age.

It's often an unfortunate side effect of prescription medications for anxiety, nerve pain, depression, and high blood
pressure. But over-the-counter drugs for allergies and colds
can dry you up as well.

Other culprits include conditions like diabetes and cancer
treatments such as radiation and chemotherapy.

Dry mouth happens when you don't have enough saliva to
keep your mouth wet, making it difficult to chew, swallow,
even talk. Without saliva to control bacteria in your mouth,
your risk of tooth decay and gum disease is higher. For
relief, try sugar-free gum and lozenges, or artificial saliva
sprays from your local drugstore.

Headaches

Do you pop a pill every time you get a headache? Stop. There are plenty of natural ways to get relief. Before you try one of them, however, you need to know what type of headache you're dealing with.

Tension. When you feel like there's a tight band wrapped around your head, with pain concentrated in your temples and forehead, it's the most common of all headaches — tension.

You may also feel clenched muscles in your neck, shoulders, and jaw, or the pain may start in the back of your head and spread forward.

Sinus. Throbbing pain in the front of your face stems from swelling in your sinuses, air-filled cavities behind your eyes, cheeks, and forehead. A sinus headache may feel worse in the morning or when you bend forward.

Migraine. If you've ever suffered a migraine, you know how crippling it can be. Severe pain on one side of your head can make you feel dizzy and nauseous. Even ordinary lights and sounds can make it worse. An aura, or group of warning symptoms, often precedes a migraine.

Cluster. That sudden, sharp pain behind one eye is called a cluster headache. It usually lasts less than an hour and happens around the same time every day.

Lots of things can trigger a headache, from stress and fatigue to skipping meals and hormonal changes in women.

No matter what the type or the cause, you don't have to grin and bear it. Check out these tried-and-true methods to heal your headaches naturally.

5 soothing solutions for your aching head

Foil head woes with a dab of oil. Forget the drugs. Tension headaches disappear like magic when you rub peppermint oil on your forehead. Don't believe it? Take a look at the research.

A solution of 10 percent peppermint oil in ethyl alcohol lowered the intensity of tension headaches after just 15 minutes, shows a study out of Germany. Researchers discovered it was just as effective as 1,000 milligrams of acetaminophen.

Some experts think peppermint oil works by relaxing the muscles around your skull or by soothing your nervous system.

To give it a go, dilute peppermint oil with alcohol before applying. The oil on its own can't penetrate your skin enough to help.

Tackle migraines with this magnificent mineral. One small mineral deficiency can leave you with fatigue, brain fog, leg cramps, mood swings — and one big headache.

People with migraines tend to have low levels of magnesium, say scientists, so they decided to put it to the test. And found magnesium supplements could cut down on the number of migraines you suffer.

How could too little magnesium cause headaches? Researchers have uncovered an important clue — the way tiny disk-shaped blood cells called platelets behave in migraine sufferers.

Platelets produce several substances your body uses for wound healing, including the hormone serotonin. But if you suffer from migraines, platelets release more serotonin than normal. Serotonin causes blood vessels to tighten up, and researchers know migraines begin just that way — with vascular constriction. Too little magnesium in your body increases serotonin, while healthy levels of the mineral help block it.

If you want to try taking supplements, keep a few cautions in mind. Men over 50 should aim for 420 milligrams (mg) daily, while women over 50 should shoot for 320 mg. Don't take more. Too much and you could experience upset stomach, diarrhea, and other tummy woes. Plus, don't take supplements at all if you have kidney disease.

Of course, you could opt for food sources, instead. Two tablespoons of chunky peanut butter will give you 30 percent of your daily requirement. An ounce of almonds, 20 percent.

Other seeds and nuts, beans, and fortified cereals will help you get a good amount of magnesium in your diet.

Drink away brain pain. It's a fact. Most people don't drink enough water. And as you get older, your body becomes less able to sense dehydration and signal your brain that you're thirsty. The bad news — becoming dehydrated may cause your head to pound.

Women who were mildly dehydrated suffered more headaches, found it more difficult to complete tasks and concentrate, and felt more tired and angry, found one study.

That's because every system in your body depends on water. When you're dehydrated, water moves out of your cells into your bloodstream in an attempt to keep your blood volume and your blood pressure at a safe level. If dehydration continues, your cells shrivel up and no longer work properly.

A common guideline is eight 8-ounce glasses of water a day. But some experts say you get much of the water you need from certain fruits and vegetables and from other beverages like milk, juice, and even caffeinated beverages like coffee, green tea, and soda.

Here are some important points to remember.

▸ Drink before you feel thirsty.

▸ Include water-rich fruits and vegetables in your diet, like berries, watermelon, grapes, peaches, tomatoes, and lettuce.

▸ Monitor your urine. Pale yellow is good. Dark amber means drink.

Massage your scalp to minimize the misery. Migraines that start at the base of your neck, at the occipital nerve, and creep up the back of your head can leave you feeling like your head's been run over by a truck. Thankfully there's something you can do that's easy and cheap.

Place a warm compress on the area for a few minutes then gently massage the base of your skull for some short-term relief.

Thwart head throbbers with popular sleep aid. For some, the sleep hormone melatonin is a miracle cure for jet lag. Could it also heal headaches? Apparently, it can.

Just 3 milligrams battled not only tension headaches but migraines as well, show two separate studies.

▸ Migraine sufferers also had fewer headaches when they took melatonin at bedtime. Over the course of the three-month study, their headaches were less intense, shorter, and didn't require pain medication as often.

▶ People who suffered chronic tension headaches an average of 20 days a month slashed those numbers down to, on average, just 13 days a month.

Melatonin could help against headaches by working as an anti-inflammatory, regulating the brain chemical dopamine and the hormone serotonin, or by hunting down toxic free radicals.

Warning

Avoid these hidden headache triggers

Could your headache woes stem from your favorite foods? You bet. Especially if you're sensitive to certain additives or ingredients.

- **Monosodium glutamate (MSG).** If your head hurts every time you eat Chinese food, it could be because of this flavor booster. Manufacturers also sprinkle it in chips, dips, soups, salad dressings, and frozen entrées.

- **Gluten.** You don't need to have celiac disease to be sensitive to gluten, the main protein in rye, wheat, and barley. Symptoms range from headaches to brain fog, joint pain to muscle cramps. Talk to your doctor about getting tested.

- **Sulfites.** Beware of these preservatives found in wine, dried fruit, vinegar, and packaged vegetables.

Knock out surprising sources of head pain

Clenching, snoring, and sneezing. What do they all have in common? The answer may surprise you — headaches. Take care of these conditions and you could find unexpected relief from chronic headache pain.

Relax your jaw. If you wake up with an aching skull, you may be grinding and clenching your teeth while you sleep. This behavior affects the area connecting your jaw to the side of your head called the temporomandibular joint. When things get bad enough, you develop temporomandibular joint disorder, commonly called TMJ. Symptoms include jaw stiffness, popping, pain, and headaches.

The cure for TMJ can be quite simple, starting with a visit to your dentist. There you can learn relaxation exercises for your jaw and get fitted for a special mouth guard to hold your jaw back and ease tension on your joint while you sleep.

Breathe and sleep easy. Morning headaches could be a sign of sleep apnea. This condition means oxygen is briefly, but frequently, cut off to your brain while you sleep. No wonder your head throbs when you get up. You can see why it's important to treat the problem and get your breathing back to normal. Two-thirds of people who had regular morning headaches also had sleep apnea, shows a Dartmouth University study.

Headaches, especially cluster headaches that disrupt your sleep, could also be due to sleep apnea. Talk to your doctor about a treatment plan.

Deal with allergies. Hay fever season is agony enough, with the runny nose, itchy eyes, and constant sneezing. Adding a migraine to the mix is like pouring salt on a wound — misery.

People who suffer from migraines have more severe headaches more often during allergy season. So treating your allergies could ease your brain pain. One study shows people who received allergy shots had half as many migraines as those who didn't get shots.

Stretch to send tension pain packing

Raise your hand if you'd rather prevent a headache than treat a headache. Who wouldn't?

A team of Italian researchers may have found a way to do just that. They tested simple, daily stretches and posture exercises on more than 900 people. After six months, the results were fewer headaches and less neck and shoulder pain. Now you can practice these same tricks yourself.

▶ Stand with your head, back, and hands against a wall. Keeping your body still, move your head forward, then pull it back until it touches the wall again. Do this eight to 10 times, every two to three hours.

▶ Take a seat in a quiet room in a comfortable chair. Apply a heating pad to your cheeks and shoulders, then relax your jaw, allowing it to drop naturally. Try this twice a day for 10 to 15 minutes at a time.

▶ Stand with your head and back against a wall. Pull your shoulders back until they touch the wall, then release them. Practice this eight to 10 times, every two to three hours.

To get the most benefit from these exercises, commit to do them every day.

Caffeine may make your headache better or worse, depending on how much you get and how often. A cup of coffee might ease a headache. But drink too much, and you could become dependent on the caffeine. Without your morning cup, you could experience the chief symptom of withdrawal — you guessed it, headache.

Hearing loss

Does it seem to you that nobody speaks clearly these days? Everyone you meet talks like "Mumbles" from the Dick Tracy movie. Or Charlie Brown's teacher. Wah, wah. You have to keep turning up the volume on the TV just to understand what they are saying — even though your spouse complains about the noise. Sound familiar? If so, listen up. You could be facing hearing loss.

Time for a sound check. If you have these symptoms, your hearing may not be up to snuff.

▸ It's difficult to understand words, and sounds seem muffled, especially in a crowd of people.

▸ You have trouble hearing consonants.

▸ You frequently ask others to slow down or speak their words more clearly.

▸ You're reluctant to participate in conversations, and you've started avoiding social gatherings.

If these symptoms sound like you, you're not alone. According to the National Institute on Deafness and Other Communication Disorders (NIDCD), one in every three adults between the ages of 65 and 74 are in the same boat. And almost half the people over 75 have some kind of hearing problem.

What type of hearing loss do you have?

Conductive hearing loss. With this condition, sound waves are not transmitted properly through your ear canal to your eardrum. This could be caused by something as simple as an ear infection, allergy, or swimmer's ear. Conductive hearing loss can often be corrected by medication or surgery.

Sensorineural hearing loss. This happens when the inner ear, or cochlea, has been damaged. Causes include head trauma, genetics, exposure to loud noises, or even simple aging. This type of loss — the most common form of permanent hearing loss — usually cannot be corrected surgically or medically.

Other factors can cause hearing loss, too, especially chronic illnesses like kidney disease, heart disease, rheumatoid arthritis, and type 2 diabetes. In fact, a recent study of more than 4,000 adults discovered even prediabetes, having higher than normal blood sugar levels without full-blown diabetes, meant a higher risk of hearing loss.

Your lifestyle can put you at risk, too. Are you a smoker? Smoking decreases the concentration of oxygen in your system, causing damage to your ears. And long-term alcohol use can harm the hair cells in your ear canal. Both might result in permanent hearing loss.

So besides using your earplugs when you've cranked up the leaf blower, what can you do to protect yourself? Here are five unexpected — but scientifically sound — ways to make sure your hearing stays clear as a bell.

Rx Alert

Your meds may hurt your ears

Here's a hidden cause of hearing loss that will shock you. More than 200 prescription and over-the-counter medications are known to cause hearing problems, reports the American Speech-Language-Hearing Association. And these ototoxic medicines, as they are called, are more common than you think. They sabotage your hearing and throw off your balance by damaging the sensory cells in your inner ear. In many cases, the effects are temporary, and things will go back to normal as soon as you stop taking the medicine. But sometimes, the damage is permanent. Be on the lookout for any new hearing problems, and report them to your doctor.

Aspirin. Taken in large doses — eight to 12 325-milligram tablets a day — aspirin may cause hearing loss or tinnitus, also known as ringing in the ears.

Other nonsteroidal anti-inflammatory drugs (NSAIDs). You know them as medicines like ibuprofen and naproxen. Studies suggest that if you take them more than twice a week, you may be putting your hearing at risk.

Acetaminophen. Taking this pain reliever — sold over the counter as brands like Tylenol — can cause hearing loss if taken more than twice per week. This is especially true if you're a man under the age of 50.

Members of the aminoglycoside antibiotic family. If you have kidney disease or a hearing problem already, you're more likely than others to suffer hearing-related side effects from antibiotics like gentamicin, streptomycin, and neomycin.

Loop diuretics. These are used to treat heart failure and high blood pressure and go by names like bumetanide (Bumex), ethacrynic acid (Edecrin), furosemide (Lasix), and torsemide (Demadex). They are most dangerous to your hearing when you take them at the same time as an aminoglycoside antibiotic.

Head off hearing loss with 4 simple tips

Take a hike to listen up. That's right. You can improve your hearing with this simple 15-minute trick.

You already know that walking is good for you. It burns calories, gives you more energy, and even helps you live longer. But scientists examining results from the famous Nurses' Health Study II have now linked a daily walk with better hearing. They found that women who walked for at least two hours a week — that's a little more than 15 minutes every day — reduced their chance of hearing loss by 15 percent, compared to women who walked less than an hour a week.

How's it work? Turns out that a little exercise, like brisk walking, increases blood flow throughout your body and ensures a good supply of oxygen. Your arteries are more likely to stay open and flexible, and by controlling weight gain, you're less likely to experience damaging inflammation to your blood vessels.

So go on. Get out there, and hear what you've been missing.

Don't worry, hear better. You probably know chronic stress can contribute to lots of serious health problems, including heart disease, diabetes, and high blood pressure. But now scientists in Sweden have discovered that stress can also hurt your ears.

Almost 10,000 people were asked questions about their sleep habits, health problems, and work stresses. By analyzing the answers, researchers found that people with the highest stress levels were most likely to suffer from hearing loss.

So how does stress affect your hearing? Thousands of tiny hairs inside your ears change noise into electrical signals that the brain translates into sounds for you. These hairs get their nutrients from your blood as it circulates through your ears.

When you get stressed, you produce lots of adrenaline — remember learning about the fight or flight response in high school biology? That extra adrenaline in your system reduces the amount of blood traveling to your inner ear. The lack of blood flow severely damages — or can even destroy — the tiny hairs, causing hearing loss.

The good news? With proper treatment and stress reduction, this type of hearing loss can sometimes be corrected. But why risk it? Take a walk, listen to music, phone a friend. Reduce your stress, save your hearing.

Foods to fix the silence. Some simple, everyday foods can help you fight hearing loss. You'll probably find just what you need, right in your kitchen.

▸ **Go fish for salmon, tuna, sardines, or trout.** The Blue Mountains Hearing Study showed that adults who ate fish twice a week lowered their chances of hearing loss by 42 percent, compared to non-fish eaters. Why? It's all about the omega-3 fatty acids. They keep you hearing loud and clear by strengthening the blood vessels in your inner ear.

▸ **Battle free radicals with antioxidants.** You can stop the damage these rogue molecules do to the nerves in your inner ear by getting healthy doses of beta carotene, vitamin C, and magnesium. A three-year study found the benefits were greatest when all these important nutrients were boosted. So eat sweet potatoes, kale, sun-dried tomatoes, spinach, and carrots — foods jam-packed with the trio.

▶ **Open a can of beans** and give your body more ammunition against the dangers of this noisy world. A B vitamin called folate may actually reduce hearing loss in seniors.

People age 50 or older who had the lowest blood levels of folate were 39 percent more likely to have hearing loss, Australian researchers discovered. They also checked blood levels of the amino acid homocysteine, because high homocysteine levels have been linked with low folate. They found that people with the highest levels of homocysteine had a 64 percent higher risk of developing hearing loss than people with normal homocysteine levels.

Low levels of folate and high levels of homocysteine can be bad news for your cochlea, a spiral-shaped chamber in your inner ear that is vital to your hearing. Your cochlea needs a good blood supply from a large number of blood vessels in order to do its job.

Unfortunately, homocysteine can damage those blood vessels. Because a shortage of folate leads to too much homocysteine, making sure you get enough folate may be a smart way to help protect your hearing. Fortunately, adding more to your diet is not hard. Lentils, pinto beans, chickpeas, black beans, and navy beans are five delicious, inexpensive, easy-to-find foods that are just brimming with it.

Musicians note better hearing as they age. Were you that child? The one who had to practice the piano every day after school while your friends played ball — and laughed at your misery? Well, guess what? The tables have turned, and you're the one who gets the last laugh. Those piano lessons have come back to help you — in a most unexpected way.

Studies show that childhood music lessons train your brain for healthy aging. As you learned to play that piano — or any musical instrument — you developed auditory skills that now help you distinguish sounds and speech. Even if you already have hearing loss, you're better at picking out sounds against a noisy background — and remembering what you heard — than those friends who practiced their fast ball instead of their scales.

It doesn't matter if you haven't tickled the ivories in years. And you don't have to be a pro like Stevie Wonder or Paul McCartney to reap the benefits. Researchers found that if you played for a decade or longer earlier in life, the brain training that came along with those music lessons will follow you all the way into old age.

Have you heard? Listening to loud music with your earbuds or headphones on could put your hearing at risk, says the World Health Organization (WHO). For safer ears, keep your volume set at less than 85 decibels — which is still as loud as a hair dryer. Power off after 60 minutes.

And it's never too late to start. So maybe you've just decided to add a little music to your life. A study conducted at the University of South Florida looked at the impact of piano lessons on adults between the ages of 60 and 85. After 16 weeks, when compared with their peers who had not taken lessons, the piano students showed improved memory, speech, and brain functions.

So blow your horn, strum your guitar, beat your drum. If you're a senior, it's music to your ears.

◀)) Dangerous decibels harm hearing ((▶

Did you know cruising down the highway in your little Deuce coupe convertible can take a toll on your ears? See how noise exposure can threaten your healthy hearing.

firecrackers, explosion, gunshot	**140***	pain and immediate ear injury possible
jackhammer, jet plane (100 ft away), stock car races	**130**	hearing loss likely in less than 1 minute
personal stereo on maximum volume	**120**	hearing loss likely in less than 1 minute
rock band, shouting in ear, chainsaw, leaf blower	**110**	hearing loss likely within 2 minutes
snowblower, diesel truck, gas lawn mower	**100**	hearing loss possible after 15 minutes
traveling the highway in a convertible, food blender	**90**	damaging after 2 hours
garbage disposal, noisy restaurant, hair dryer	**80**	unsafe only after lengthy exposure
city traffic, washing machine, normal speech, alarm clock	**70**	annoying but safe for adults

*Noise level in decibels

Get the wax out — safely

Your ears are designed to clean themselves. Whenever you eat or speak, the movement of your lower jaw pushes earwax toward your outer ear. But when a lot of earwax is produced — usually in older people — it can form a plug in your ear canal that impairs your hearing.

Use these tips to clean your ears. But not the cotton kind. Cotton swabs can push the wax further into your ear canal.

- Soften the earwax by applying a few drops of olive, baby, or mineral oil into your ear canal twice a day for up to five days.

- Once the earwax has softened — usually after a day or two — use a rubber-bulb syringe to gently squirt lukewarm water into your ear canal. To do this, first tilt your head. Then pull your outer ear up and back to straighten the ear canal.

- When finished, turn your head to the side so the water can drain out.

- Dry your ear with a soft towel.

- Repeat the flushing steps as needed.

Heartburn

The smell of your favorite foods wafting through the house is enough to brighten anybody's day — unless you're prone to heartburn. Instead, all you can think about is whether or not that meal will come back to haunt you later.

Most people experience the occasional bout of heartburn — a burning sensation behind your breastbone, a cough, or trouble swallowing. It can be caused by certain foods, medications, or just overeating. But if you get chronic heartburn, you have a condition called gastroesophageal reflux disease (GERD).

Heartburn happens when stomach acid flows back into your esophagus, the tube that carries food and liquid from your mouth to your stomach. There's a muscle that's supposed to keep them separate, called the lower esophageal sphincter. If you have GERD this muscle is weak, so it can't stop the flow of acid.

If GERD goes untreated, the acid backwash can cause long-term damage to your esophagus and trigger cell mutations that lead to esophageal cancer. Fortunately, most people are able to stop the pain with a few simple lifestyle adjustments.

Find your triggers. When it comes to figuring out what's causing your heartburn, round up the usual suspects. Chocolate, spicy food, salt, fried food, garlic, and acidic foods like citrus and tomatoes are common culprits. But everybody reacts to foods differently, so try eliminating certain items from your diet to see if your symptoms clear up.

How you eat matters, too. Even if you're making healthy food choices, bad meal habits could cause indigestion and heartburn.

When heartburn pain is a frequent guest at your table, here are some things you can try.

▶ **Eat less, more often.** Smaller meals, four to six times a day are better than two or three big ones.

▶ **Ban late-night snacking.** In fact, you shouldn't even lie down for four hours after you eat.

▶ **Slim down.** If you're overweight, losing those extra pounds might be the answer. The extra weight squeezes your belly and forces stomach acid up your windpipe.

5 hot tips to cool down heartburn

Position your pillow to relieve the pain. Your pillow is more than just a place to rest your head — it's the secret weapon to beating several health problems, especially heartburn. To fight nighttime problems with GERD, pick up a wedge-shaped foam pillow. It will raise your esophagus so the acid can't escape your stomach. If that's not comfortable, tuck the wedge behind your back and train yourself to sleep on your left side. This helps clear the acid out of your esophagus.

Here are three more ways your pillow can help you get the shut-eye you deserve.

▶ **Relax a backache.** Sleeping on your back puts heavy pressure on your spine. Place a pillow under your knees to take this pressure off. For even more relief, sleep on your side with a pillow between your knees.

▶ **Fend off leg cramps.** Use an extra pillow to prop your feet up, if leg cramps keep you awake. This keeps your calf muscles lengthened and blood from pooling in your feet.

▶ **Tame neck pain.** Do you constantly wake with a crick in your neck? Then your pillow may be tilting your head while you sleep. Find a pillow that keeps your head in a neutral position.

H2O can douse those flames. Water can smother fires and put out heartburn pain. One study found that drinking water reduced stomach acid in just one minute.

Even better, drinking water throughout the day protects you from flare-ups by keeping your esophagus clear of acid. Just be careful not to drink too much, especially with meals. Water can dilute the contents of your stomach, making it harder to digest your food. Try to avoid drinking for an hour before or after you eat.

High-fiber foods fight the fire inside. Make high-fiber breads your new "go-to" if you have gastroesophageal reflux disease (GERD) with its frequent bouts of heartburn and indigestion.

A Norwegian study found people who regularly ate high-fiber breads essentially sliced their risk of GERD in half, compared to those who preferred low-fiber white bread.

Experts think fiber may work by scavenging nitrites in the stomach, lowering the amount of nitric oxide produced. Nitric oxide may relax the lower esophageal sphincter, leading to acid reflux.

Work out your jaw to keep heartburn at bay. The more you chew, the more saliva you produce. And with the compounds in saliva that neutralize stomach acid, that means less acid reflux. So make sure to chew your food slowly and thoroughly. For extra protection from heartburn, chew a piece of sugar-free gum after eating.

Enjoy coffee again with this simple swap. There's hope for you if you love java, but hate the heartburn that comes with it. It could be as simple as switching from a light-roast coffee to a dark one.

Experts say dark-roasted coffee contains double the amount of N-methylpyridinium (NMP), a compound that helps reduce stomach acid.

Just bear in mind caffeine triggers the secretion of stomach acid. Your best bet is a decaffeinated, dark-roasted coffee.

Rx Alert

Bad medicine?
When heartburn hurts your bones

A particular type of heartburn medicine known as proton pump inhibitors (PPIs) makes you more likely to fracture a hip.

One study shows postmenopausal women who took PPIs for at least two years were 35 percent more likely to suffer a hip fracture, especially if they smoked. What's more, the longer they took them, the higher their risk. Women who took these drugs for six to eight years raised their risk to 55 percent.

Scientists say PPIs may disrupt bone growth and calcium absorption in your body. They may also lower bone mineral density by wreaking havoc on your thyroid.

All is not lost though if you've been on heartburn meds for awhile. Two years after the women in the study stopped taking them, their hip fracture risk dropped back to normal.

If you take medications like these, talk to your doctor, but don't stop taking them on your own.

- omeprazole (Prilosec)
- esomeprazole (Nexium)
- lansoprazole (Prevacid)
- rabeprazole (Aciphex)
- pantoprazole (Protonix)
- dexlansoprazole (Kapidex)

Kitchen herbs to sweeten your sour stomach

Sometimes your problem isn't just heartburn, but a severe bout of indigestion, with symptoms like bloating, nausea, pain, or burping. Instead of reaching for costly medications, give these 10 healing herbs a try. They may work as well as drugs to soothe tummy woes and get your digestive system back on track.

Basil. Every time you cook with basil, you're adding an herb chock-full of antioxidant, antibacterial, and anti-inflammatory properties to your meal. What's more, you can use it to treat gas and lack of appetite.

Caraway. You'll find them in rye bread and many popular German dishes like sauerkraut, but caraway seeds are also used to relieve a variety of gastrointestinal problems. Sprinkle them into a pot of beans or cabbage. They'll crank up the flavor and crank down that embarrassing side effect — gas.

Chamomile. A tea made from chamomile calms everything from stomach cramps to indigestion and irritable bowel syndrome. Scientists think it helps by relaxing muscles that move food through your intestines, getting rid of gas, and soothing your stomach.

Cinnamon. You know cinnamon adds an aromatic punch to pies, cobblers, and other treats. But did you know this humble spice can relieve indigestion? That's what practitioners of old-time medicine have known for years.

Ayurvedic and traditional Chinese medicine make use of cinnamon to treat digestive disorders, including indigestion, gas, and diarrhea. Ancient Greeks and Romans also used cinnamon for better digestion. Even today, it's recommended by herbalists and approved in Germany to soothe indigestion, bloating, and gas

Although scientists can't tell you how it works, it might have to do with the way cinnamon warms up your stomach and helps stimulate digestion.

While there have been few human studies to support the medicinal use of cinnamon, it can't hurt to add a few dashes of this delightful spice to your meals. Try sprinkling ground cinnamon on cooked carrots, winter squash, sweet potatoes, or your morning oatmeal. Or swizzle cinnamon sticks in hot cider, coffee drinks, or juices.

Coriander (cilantro). Not only does this herb help curb IBS symptoms, scientists believe coriander contains chemicals that help absorb and get rid of gas.

Fennel. Nibbling from a dish of aromatic fennel seeds is an age-old remedy for indigestion and gas. The secret may be the phytochemical anethole, a compound that relaxes your stomach muscles, speeds up digestion, and prompts your liver to make more bile. Herbal experts say these effects can help flatten a bloated belly; relieve indigestion, stomachache, and heartburn; and may even ease diarrhea, constipation, and irritable bowel syndrome symptoms. Fennel seeds also make a tasty addition to soups, pastas, and roasted veggies.

Ginger. Thanks to its natural chemicals, ginger is not only an anti-nausea powerhouse, it triggers movement in your digestive tract, protects your stomach lining, keeps you regular, and breaks up gas. Add it to those gas-producing foods for a zingy taste.

Parsley. When you need gas relief, reach for parsley. This highly nutritional herb calms gas cramps with a pleasing side effect — it freshens your breath, too.

Peppermint. Nothing beats peppermint for irritable bowel syndrome (IBS). People with IBS who took 225 milligrams of peppermint oil in a capsule showed better improvement over those who took a placebo. Peppermint may also help with gas, nausea, diarrhea, indigestion, and constipation. Just beware, it can make your heartburn worse.

Rosemary. Antioxidants, phytonutrients, and essential fatty acids — they're all in this wonderfully fragrant herb you can cook with to tackle indigestion.

Warning

Don't dismiss chest pain — it could be deadly

Your esophagus is right behind your heart. So is that pain indigestion or a heart attack? Heart attack symptoms are often milder than expected, especially in women. That means you shouldn't take any chances. Call for medical help immediately if you experience:

- pain that radiates to your left arm, shoulder, jaw, or neck.

- shortness of breath.

- sweating, restlessness, or anxiety.

- nausea.

- pressure in your chest.

Heart disease

Uncle Jim had a heart attack. Grandma is recovering from a stroke. Your dad suffers from angina. Their conditions may be different, but they all suffer from the same thing — heart disease. And you'd better watch out because the future could hold the same for you.

Heart disease is a term that covers problems ranging from a weak heart muscle and abnormal heartbeat to valve disorders and even infections. By far, the most common problem area is your arteries. The technical name — cardiovascular disease — usually refers to conditions that involve narrowed or blocked blood vessels. They are often the source of these serious conditions:

▸ **Angina.** Ever had chest pain? It could be caused by reduced blood flow to the heart.

▸ **Heart failure.** The tricky term actually means your heart doesn't pump blood as well as it should.

▸ **Peripheral artery disease.** Narrowed blood vessels reduce blood flow to your limbs.

▸ **Heart attack.** If narrow arteries and plaque block blood flow to the heart, the tissue could die.

▸ **Stroke.** When clogged arteries cut off blood flow to your brain, it can suffer severe damage.

▸ **Aneurysm.** A bulge in the wall of a weakened blood vessel can burst and cause internal bleeding.

▶ **Sudden cardiac arrest.** Your heart stops beating unexpectedly.

A family history of heart problems puts you at high risk. While you can't change genetics or other risk factors like growing older or being male, you do have control over many things that contribute to heart disease. Experts think more than 200,000 people could be saved each year if they managed health risks by changing certain habits.

By the time you finish reading this chapter, an estimated 17 Americans will have died from heart disease. You don't have to be one of them. Lower your risk and give yourself a fighting chance by learning the secrets of a healthy heart.

5 simple steps keep your ticker in top shape

Strengthen your heart from the ground up — with plants. Years ago, researchers asked an important question. Can you stop heart disease without medication? What they discovered could change your life.

The secret, they found, is a plant-based diet. In fact, healthy habits and a vegetarian diet may actually reverse coronary artery disease in just a year.

New research agrees that plants have the power. Scientists looked at the eating habits of more than 400,000 European volunteers. Those who favored plant-based foods and less meat had a 20 percent lower risk of dying from heart disease than the heavy meat eaters.

Why are plant-based diets so good? It's a combo of adding more nutrients from plant foods and taking out harmful ingredients found in animal products, especially processed meats. Sodium, nitrates, and L-carnitine are some examples. Eating a lot of red meat actually raises your risk of dying from heart disease, says a study published in *The American Journal of Clinical Nutrition*.

But don' t worry — you won't have to become a vegetarian to snag the benefits. Just eating more plant foods will do your body good. Limit meat to twice a week, and you'll help avoid high blood sugar, blood pressure, cholesterol, and even excess belly fat.

'Miraculous' diet reverses biggest health woes

Who knew?

What if someone told you two foods could significantly reverse your risk of heart failure? All you have to do is follow the diet people have called "little short of miraculous."

The Kempner rice diet, named after its founder, originally consisted of rice and fruit — a drastic eating plan that has helped people when nothing else could.

Today, the food selection is a little more appetizing. It has been expanded to include rice, grains, fruits, vegetables and beans, with an option of occasional fish. The goal of these powerful plant foods is to get people off medication and reverse their life-threatening conditions.

When you take out salt, fat, cholesterol, and animal protein, you eliminate common contributors to high blood pressure, kidney disease, and heart disease. This gives your body the chance to heal and reverse damage.

Since it's such a restrictive diet, you'll need a doctor to monitor your progress. For more information, go online to *ricehouse.org*, or call 919-220-5646.

Sit less, move more. Aaron hits the gym every day. He thinks a 30-minute, heart-pounding workout is enough to keep his ticker in good condition. What he doesn't know is sitting at work all day and lounging around watching TV all night might be canceling out his hard work.

"Regardless of how much physical activity someone gets, prolonged sedentary time could negatively impact the health of your heart and blood vessels," says Deborah Rohm Young, Ph.D., chair of a paper on sedentary behavior published by the American Heart Association.

That means your weekly workouts may not balance out the hours you spend browsing the internet, reading a new book, or driving to work. But adding more activity to your leisure time can lower your risk of heart disease and heart-related death, Young says.

So don't fall victim to "sitting disease." Get off the couch and spend more time doing those things you already love, such as gardening, walking, dancing, or fishing. And try to add a little activity when you're desk-bound or watching your favorite show, even if it's just stretching or walking around the room. Every little bit helps your heart.

Control the big four that supercharge your risk. What's the first thing that happens at the doctor's office? The nurse probably weighs you and takes your blood pressure. That's because problems on the scale and under the cuff can lead to problems everywhere. In fact, abnormal numbers in any of these categories supercharge your risk of heart disease.

> ▸ **Weight.** Drop your risk of heart disease by maintaining your midriff. Your Body Mass Index (BMI) should be less than 25.

▸ **Blood pressure.** High BP can sabotage your arteries. Aim for numbers below 120/80 mmHg.

▸ **Cholesterol.** Too much bad cholesterol can block your arteries and increase your risk of heart attack and stroke. Keep total cholesterol less than 200 mg/dL.

▸ **Blood sugar.** Glucose causes blood vessels to constrict, says recent research. This can raise blood pressure, limit the flow of nutrients, and make a heart attack more severe. Keep your blood sugar level less than 100 mg/dL.

Warning

The not-so-sweet truth — sugar has a sour side

You put a dollar bill into a vending machine and out come 10 packs of sugar. You would never eat all those, right? Well, you drink just as much every time you toss back a can of soda. And all that sugar comes with a price. What's the damage? Higher odds of heart disease and stroke, studies say.

Most women shouldn't eat more than 100 calories of added sugar a day, says the American Heart Association. Men can safely get about 50 calories more. That means just one Classic coke could be enough to push you over.

And switching to diet soda won't help. The artificial sweeteners used in diet drinks are also linked to heart damage. Plus, they crank up cravings for sweets.

You can tame the sugar monster with a two-week challenge to reset your taste buds. Simply cut out added sugars and artificial sweeteners for 14 days. Bye bye cravings.

Ditch dicey habits that hurt your heart. Cigarettes and booze are two health-robbing habits you need to kick if you want to keep your ticker in tip-top shape.

▶ They're called "coffin nails" and "cancer sticks" for a reason — cigarettes put you on the fast track to all kinds of health problems. And it's not just lung disease and cancer you have to worry about. Smoking also lands you in the heart disease danger zone.

It's easy to see why. When you breathe in smoke, toxins flood your body, starving your organs of oxygen and making your heart pump harder. Just a few puffs can bump up blood pressure and make it easier for blood to clot. No wonder smokers suffer a higher risk of clogged arteries and stroke than those who "just say no."

▶ Alcohol is a less obvious threat to your heart. You thought it was supposed to protect it, right? Studies show this may be true for some heart conditions but not all. A sobering review published in the *Journal of the American College of Cardiology* says drinking alcohol, even in moderation, can lead to a higher risk of atrial fibrillation (AFib), or irregular heartbeat.

"People who continue to consume alcohol at moderate rates may notice their irregular heartbeats become more frequent," says lead study author Dr. Peter M. Kistler. "This is concerning, because it can lead to serious issues such as heart failure and stroke." Kistler says people with AFib should have no more than one alcoholic drink per day with two alcohol-free days a week. Better yet — give it up altogether.

Smog and smoke — new risk for stroke

Sound the alarm. A shocking source has just been ranked one of the top 10 causes of stroke.

Scientists already know air pollution is linked to damage in your lungs, heart, and brain. But they were surprised to learn about a third of strokes can be chalked up to impure air.

They suspect toxins that breeze about big cities cause inflammation and oxidative stress. These two terrors trigger changes in your arteries and raise blood pressure.

"People should limit their exposure on days with higher air pollution levels," says scientist Tao Liu, Ph.D., "especially those with high blood pressure."

Check *AirNow.gov* to find out the quality of your outdoor air. And remember, it's not all about outside. Cooking fumes, fireplace smoke, and chemicals can contribute to bad air quality. To clear the air under your roof, try an air purifier, run an exhaust fan in your bathroom and kitchen, and replace old wood stoves.

De-stress your life to fight inflammation. Can you die of a broken heart? That's what many people suspected when Debbie Reynolds died just one day after her daughter Carrie Fisher. While it's true that extreme physical or emotional strain can temporarily stun your heart, everyday stress can cause heart troubles, too.

Anxiety doesn't just bump up cholesterol and spike your blood pressure. A new study is the first to discover a surprising connection between your brain, your heart, and your worries.

Activity in the amygdala — an area of the brain involved in emotions like fear — is linked to inflammation in your arteries. Researchers found that, out of almost 300 people, those with more action in their amygdalas had a greater risk of heart disease and stroke.

Protect your heart by forcing yourself to unwind whenever your stress levels rise. Take slow deep breaths, go for a walk in nature, listen to classical music, or play with your pup.

Ward off heart attack and stroke the Mediterranean way

The Mediterranean diet is one of the hottest eating plans in America — and one of the most highly recommended for fighting heart disease. But what makes it so good for your ticker? This delicious diet is chock-full of nutrients that help your heart, even if you're at high risk for heart troubles.

To test it out, researchers recruited more than 7,000 people between the ages of 55 and 80 who were in the high-risk category. They advised one group to lower the amount of fat they were eating. The other two groups adopted a Mediterranean diet supplemented with either extra-virgin olive oil or tree nuts.

The result? The Mediterranean diet plans lowered the risk of dying from heart attack or stroke by 30 percent. Quite an accomplishment. And heart benefits aren't the only perks of this eating plan. The following 12 Mediterranean diet staples also work like medicines against diabetes, arthritis, dementia, vision loss, and sleep problems.

Olive oil and walnuts.
Leave artery-clogging
saturated fats at the store
and bring home more
unsaturated varieties. Your
arteries will thank you.

The American Heart Association suggests you reduce
saturated fat to about 7 percent of total calories if your
cholesterol levels are good; 5
percent if LDL cholesterol is
high. For a man eating
2,000 calories a day, 5 percent equals about 11 grams
of saturated fat — the amount found in one Burger King
Whopper. Add cheese and you're already over. Instead, go for
heart-healthy unsaturated fats found in olive oil and walnuts.

Do you often wonder if you should be taking aspirin? Here's the scoop. If you've had heart problems, you'll benefit from aspirin's blood-thinning abilities. Follow your doctor's advice. But if you have no history of heart disease, you may be better off without it. The risk of bleeding often outweighs potential benefits.

Lentils and oats. Eating more fiber may prevent strokes, reveals
an analysis of eight long-term studies. Scientists found that
increasing fiber by 7 grams a day was linked to a 7 percent
reduction in stroke risk. You'll easily get that much from a half
cup of cooked lentils or a half cup of oats.

Potatoes and prunes. What do spuds and dried plums have in
common? They're both loaded with potassium. This "miracle"
mineral brings down blood pressure, and research says that's
only the tip of the iceberg.

A 12-year study showed you can reduce your chance of having a
deadly stroke up to a whopping 40 percent simply by adding
more potassium-rich foods to your meals.

Flaxseed and fatty fish. Looking for a simple way to lower your risk of heart disease? Eat more omega-3 fatty acids, say Penn State nutritionists. This nutrient helps support healthy arteries and lower high blood pressure. Whether you get omega-3 from fish or flaxseed, your arteries will be happy and relaxed.

Blackberries and spinach. Berries and leafy greens are packed with vitamins that act as antioxidants, hunting down dangerous free radicals. Antioxidants in fruits, vegetables, whole grains, and coffee help fend off heart attack and stroke, says a study published in *The American Journal of Medicine*.

Yogurt and chocolate. The probiotics in yogurt can lower risk factors associated with heart disease, particularly high LDL cholesterol levels, high blood pressure, and inflammation. But the news gets even better. Probiotics dine on indigestible fiber called prebiotics — and dark chocolate turns out to be a good source.

"The good microbes, such as *Bifidobacterium* and lactic acid bacteria, feast on chocolate," says researcher Maria Moore. "When you eat dark chocolate, they grow and ferment it, producing compounds that are anti-inflammatory." Defending your heart against inflammation helps lower your risk of stroke.

Give the Mediterranean diet a try, and see how well this delicious meal plan works for you. You just might feel like shouting "Opa!"

The magic elixir that helps your arteries clean themselves

You've got what you need to keep your arteries clean as a whistle, and it's just on the other side of your pantry door. At only a nickel per ounce, vinegar could be the cheapest way to lower blood pressure naturally and prevent heart disease.

How your heart's "highway" gets congested. An intricate system of blood vessels flows throughout your body, from just below the surface of your skin to the deepest parts of your organs. Picture the interstates that crisscross America, and you'll get a good idea of the complex network inside your body.

When you eat a meal high in trans and saturated fats, it raises the level of low-density lipoprotein (LDL) cholesterol in your bloodstream. LDL is seen as "bad" because it deposits cholesterol into your arteries. Eat enough burgers and fries, and all that cholesterol will stick together and clog your arteries, like a fleet of 18-wheelers blocking the interstate.

The more bad fats you eat, the bigger the pileup, until one day you can no longer squeeze your little red Corvette through the congestion. That's when heart disease sets in. Fatty deposits streak your vessels from head to toe, causing your blood pressure to spike as your blood fights to get through the blockages.

Clear out the traffic jams in your arteries. The interesting thing is, if you eat a salad with vinaigrette dressing along with those burgers, you may protect your arteries from the effects of those bad fats. Turns out the vinegar in that dressing is a powerful artery cleanser, and here's why.

▸ Vinegar boosts the enzyme that triggers the production of nitric oxide in your arteries, Japanese scientists have found. Nitric oxide relaxes your blood vessels, which causes them to widen and allow blood to flow freely. The researchers measured blood flow in postmenopausal women and found those who had taken a tablespoon of vinegar beforehand had better blood flow than a placebo group. They believe it's the acetic acid in vinegar that delivers this artery-healing benefit.

▶ Balsamic vinegar boosts the heart-healthy benefits above and beyond other vinegars, suggests another Japanese study. Balsamic vinegar is made from grapes, which are loaded with natural compounds called polyphenols. These powerful compounds put the brakes on LDL oxidation, which contributes to inflammation in your arteries.

Add a little vinegar to your menu every day, and you'll arm yourself with another valuable weapon in your battle against heart disease.

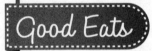

Sneak vinegar into your daily diet

A tablespoon a day is all it takes to reap the heart-healthy rewards of vinegar. Don't drink it straight as it can burn your esophagus. Instead, try these simple and delicious tricks.

- Mix vinegar in with rice or potato salad.

- Stir it into drinks and smoothies.

- Make vinaigrettes for your green salads.

- Dip chunks of whole-grain bread into balsamic vinegar.

- Try specially flavored vinegars like peach and passion fruit over cold pasta salads.

Saunas — the hottest therapy for your heart

"The sauna is a poor man's pharmacy," goes an old Finnish saying. The Finns understood how the warmth of a sauna can rejuvenate you both mentally and physically. But who would have thought it could actually cut your risk for heart attack and stroke?

In a 20-year study surveying more than 2,000 Finnish men, researchers compared volunteers who reported one sauna session each week with those who were in the sauna four to seven times a week. Amazingly, the risk of death from heart disease was cut in half for the frequent users, especially for those whose "sweat sessions" lasted more than 19 minutes.

Hot water baths also seem to be protective, say Japanese researchers who studied hot spring therapy.

Many factors may contribute to heat's positive effects on your cardiovascular system, scientists say. Here are a few.

▶ High temperatures activate heat shock proteins that help reduce oxidative stress and inflammation in your arteries. These stabilizing proteins also increase nitric oxide, which signals the muscles in your blood vessels to relax. As stiff arteries loosen up, blood flow improves and your blood pressure drops.

▶ A session in the sauna raises your heart rate as much as low-to-moderate-intensity exercise. So you actually reap some of the benefits of exercise while sitting around chatting with your friends. And that time spent relaxing and socializing may also contribute to the sauna's beneficial effects.

Talk to your doctor to find out if it's safe for you to try heat therapy. Saunas, hot baths, and showers might be fine depending on your health, the temperature, and how long you bathe. If he gives you the go-ahead, build up your time gradually, and watch out for signs of overheating, such as nausea and dizziness.

Rx Alert

NSAIDs linked to heart failure

Do you take nonsteroidal anti-inflammatory drugs (NSAIDs) like ibuprofen or naproxen? If so, you may be at higher risk for heart failure — even if you've never had problems. That's what a new study revealed after evaluating almost 10 million NSAID users.

These drugs are often prescribed to treat pain and inflammation. But according to research published in *The BMJ*, side effects may outweigh the benefits.

Current use of any of the 27 NSAIDs included in the study led to a 19 percent higher risk for heart failure, compared to past use. Sound alarming? It is.

Heart failure occurs when your heart doesn't pump blood as well as it should, leading to fluid buildup in your body. The resulting symptoms could land you in the hospital. In fact, people who took the following nine NSAIDs were most likely to be admitted for heart failure.

- diclofenac
- ibuprofen
- indomethacin
- ketorolac
- naproxen
- nimesulide
- piroxicam
- etoricoxib
- rofecoxib

Higher doses also increased the likelihood of an ailing heart. Some NSAIDs could actually double your risk if taken at a very high dose. Talk to your doctor if you take any of the medications listed.

High blood pressure

Your heart is the hardest working muscle in your body, pumping about 2,000 gallons of blood every day. You certainly don't want to make its job any harder. But that's exactly what happens when you clog up your arteries by smoking, sitting all day, eating the wrong foods, and engaging in other unhealthy habits.

Imagine how hard it would be to drink a smoothie if you pinched the straw between your fingers. Likewise, when blood vessels are blocked, your heart has to work extra hard to get oxygen and nutrients where they need to be.

Many problems start when plaque builds up on artery walls as a response to damage and inflammation. Doctors call this atherosclerosis. Over time, the plaque can harden, stiffening and narrowing arteries so blood can't pass through properly. That increases the pressure on your artery walls. If the pressure stays high, it's known as hypertension, or high blood pressure.

You may never have any symptoms, but that doesn't mean your body isn't suffering silently. If blood is blocked from cells downstream, it can result in a host of serious problems — and not only for your heart.

▸ **Brain damage.** Like a kink in a water hose, high blood pressure can cause an artery to burst. Or it can block an artery so that too little blood gets to the brain, causing a stroke.

▶ **Kidney disease.** Damaged blood vessels in your kidneys are a disaster waiting to happen. If they're not healthy, they eventually stop removing wastes, toxins, and extra fluid from your bloodstream. And a buildup of fluid raises your blood pressure even more, which further damages your kidneys. Diabetes is the No. 1 cause of kidney failure in the United States. But coming in at No. 2? You got it — high blood pressure.

▶ **Vision loss.** Strain on the tiny blood vessels in your eyes can wreak havoc on your retina and optic nerve.

One out of three Americans has blood pressure that is consistently too high. Are you one of them? Here's how to tell. When you check your blood pressure, you'll see two numbers. The top number, systolic, measures the force of blood against artery walls as your heart beats. The lower number, diastolic, measures the force between beats.

Experts usually encourage folks to get their blood pressure below 120/80 mmHg. Doing this would save more than 100,000 lives each year in the United States, they say.

While you may eventually need medication to control your high blood pressure, diet and lifestyle changes can ease the strain on your ticker and bring down your numbers naturally.

Lower your blood pressure with 12 'heart'y habits

Sprinkle on seeds to help your blood flow smoothly. Coat your frying pan with cooking spray and your food will slide right off. Would you believe you can get the same slippery effect in your arteries? The secret is alpha-linolenic acid (ALA), an essential fatty acid that coats your arteries like a nonstick spray, keeping your blood flowing smoothly.

One of the best sources of ALA is the tiny flaxseed. This miracle food has a trio of heart healthy benefits. It helps protect against high blood pressure, high cholesterol, and heart disease. And it even helps fight obesity.

Along with ALA, these little seeds contain insoluble fiber and potent antioxidants called lignans. And sneaking a little into your diet each day is easy.

In one study, volunteers ate foods like bagels, muffins, buns, and pasta containing about 2 tablespoons of ground flaxseed every day. These volunteers had peripheral artery disease, which is related to hardened, narrow arteries. But in six months, their systolic blood pressure dropped about 10 mmHg, and their diastolic blood pressure went down about 7 mmHg.

Here's the best news. A 10-point improvement in the top number could lower your risk for stroke by 36 percent and heart attack by 27 percent. Plus, a seven-point dip in the bottom number might have a similar effect on stroke and heart disease. Who knew a tiny seed could have such a big impact?

Gain a school of benefits from a single nutrient. Big things sometimes come in small packages. Take the tiny sardine. It may be small, but this fish is loaded with memory-saving vitamin D and fatigue-fighting CoQ10, not to mention heart-healing omega-3 fatty acids. Plus it stimulates weight loss. It's one delicious, nutrition-packed food you're probably not eating, but should be.

Omega 3 fatty acids are a big deal because they reduce inflammation and lower the risk of chronic illnesses like heart disease. Your body can't make omega-3 fatty acids, so you have to get them from food. Luckily, there are plenty of fish in the sea.

You may not have considered sardines, but they're a superb choice because they have very little mercury, a toxin found in many fatty fish. But you can also get your omega-3 from mackerel, salmon, and albacore tuna.

The heart benefits are no fish tale. A study in *The Journal of Nutrition* shows that two to three servings of oily fish each week lowers systolic blood pressure by 5 mmHg in folks who have high blood pressure. That could cut your risk for heart disease by 20 percent.

Not only is this tasty food good for your heart, it also helps prevent Alzheimer's, belly fat, diabetes — even wrinkles. With all its benefits, you may want to include it in your diet every day.

Don't have a heart for fish? Get omega-3 from walnuts, flaxseeds, soybeans, pumpkin seeds, and more.

Clean your arteries with a delicious garden favorite. In 1893, the big debate was settled. According to the Supreme Court, tomatoes would be classified as vegetables. Of course, you may not care what they're called as long as you can enjoy their juicy tang on your latest sandwich masterpiece.

But culinary creations are not all they're good for. Tomatoes are actually a blessing to your blood pressure. Why? Because this artery-cleaning veggie acts like a scrub brush to clean out cholesterol and reduce high blood pressure.

Your arteries get in trouble when LDL cholesterol in your blood becomes oxidized and sticks to artery walls. It builds up to form plaque, which clogs your arteries. Your heart then has to pump harder to get the blood from point A to point B. Tomatoes help because they're a rich source of lycopene, an antioxidant that keeps your cholesterol from oxidizing.

What's your favorite way to eat tomatoes? If you love them crushed up in marinara sauce over a big plate of spaghetti, you're on the right track. Lycopene seems to help best when tomatoes are cooked. So go ahead and pour some sauce over your pasta or add a cup of low-sodium tomato juice to your breakfast routine.

Slash high BP risk in half in a few smooth moves. Did you know that fidgeting while you watch your favorite show gets your blood moving enough to protect your arteries? If tapping your toes can do that, imagine what you could do if you went for a stroll every day.

It's no secret — walking and other activities are a bonus for your blood pressure. And recently, scientists put it to the test in an interesting way. They looked at more than 1,000 people who moved to neighborhoods with better access to grocery stores, restaurants, banks, and other shops within walking distance.

They found that people who moved from a car-dependent city to a walking-friendly neighborhood were better off. In fact, they were 54 percent less likely to have high blood pressure compared to folks who moved to another neighborhood that required a car to run errands.

You don't have to sell your home to get these great benefits. Form an exercise group to keep you motivated, or walk solo at a nearby mall or park. Aim to get moving for at least 30 minutes every day.

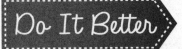

Get a grip: simple way to squeeze out high blood pressure

Want to add a boost to your exercise routine? Crush high blood pressure with isometric hand grippers.

It's unsurprising that experts give grippers two thumbs up. They were first studied in the 60s, when scientists noticed a trend. Fighter pilots training with hand-grip exercises to keep from blacking out during turns and dives had lower blood pressure.

A recent study showed that hand-grip exercises helped drop systolic blood pressure 10 points and diastolic pressure five points over 10 weeks.

You can easily find hand grippers online or at your local sporting goods store and try them yourself. Just squeeze for three minutes and rest five minutes. Repeat five times. Do this three days a week, and you'll be on your way to better blood pressure.

Steady sodium levels with a mighty mineral. Mr. Potato Head is just a toy, but if he could talk, he'd tell you that real spuds can drop your blood pressure like a hot potato. Red, white, and sweet potatoes are splendid, but the best may be the one that doesn't often make it to the table — the purple potato.

Colorful plant foods are chock-full of healthy phytochemicals, and so it is with the potato. Eating six to eight small purple spuds twice a day for a month was all it took for folks to lower their blood pressure. And even though most people were already taking medication, both systolic and diastolic blood pressure dropped another four to five points.

You may be surprised to learn the potato is packed with pressure-balancing ingredients like fiber, magnesium, calcium, kukoamines, and potassium. And of all of them, potassium is the most critical because of its unique relationship with sodium.

Sodium can make your body hang on to fluids, forcing your heart to pump harder to get the added volume through your blood vessels. When this happens, potassium steps in and tells your kidneys to excrete more sodium and fluids to relieve the pressure on your artery walls.

To make sure you're keeping your sodium levels — and your blood pressure — in balance, eat more high-potassium foods like prunes, raisins, lima beans, and bananas.

Relax your arteries with a tangy tea. Looking for a delicious way to lower blood pressure? This brew does it better than even some medications, studies say.

▸ Researchers found that two cups of strong hibiscus tea each morning lowered blood pressure as well as a starting dose of captopril, a leading blood-pressure medication.

▸ Three cups of hibiscus tea every day for six weeks lowered blood pressure in volunteers by seven points, says a study published in *The Journal of Nutrition*.

Scientists think the active ingredient in hibiscus, *H. sabdariffa*, may relax and widen arteries and also act as a diuretic to help your body eliminate extra water and salt.

Although hibiscus is an exotic flower, you don't have to go far to find it. Look for teas with its deliciously tart, cranberry-like flavor in stores and online.

Warning

How low can you go? Dangers of driving down blood pressure

You've been working hard to get your blood pressure down, and it's finally under 120 mmHg like your doctor recommended. Before you paint the town red, take a peek at the bottom number. If it's too low, you may be at risk for heart damage.

For years, doctors were happy if you kept your systolic pressure in the 130 to 140 range. Then a large study called the Systolic Blood Pressure Intervention Trial (SPRINT) found that getting your numbers down to 120/80 significantly lowered the risk of both fatal and nonfatal heart problems. That goal became the new golden standard.

Recently, however, researchers at Johns Hopkins School of Medicine discovered that ultra-low blood pressure is just as harmful as high blood pressure. In fact, diastolic BP below 60 mmHg is linked to a higher risk of heart disease and death from any cause. Their recommendation? Keep your bottom number above 70.

The nut that battles artery-damaging stress. Have you ever heard of the "happy nut"? That's what the Chinese call the pistachio, whose nickname comes from the small, grin-like crack in the shell. But research reveals a whole new reason to smile. These tasty nuts improve your blood pressure by relaxing blood vessels and supporting the inner lining, which may help lower your risk for heart disease.

A Penn State study supported by the American Pistachio Growers shows people with type 2 diabetes may especially benefit from eating pistachios. Researchers measured participants' blood pressure during a stressful situation. They either put a hand in cold water for two and a half minutes or performed challenging math problems.

"After the pistachio diet, blood vessels remained more relaxed and open during the stress tests," says Sheila G. West, professor of biobehavioral health and nutritional sciences.

The results are not as nutty as they sound. Your heart beats faster as stress and anxiety pile up. That spikes your blood pressure, which puts a bigger load on your heart. But eating half a cup to a cup of pistachios a day may calm your body's response to daily stress.

"Although nuts are high in fat, they contain good fats, fiber, potassium, and antioxidants," says West. "Given the high risk of heart disease in people with diabetes, nuts are an important part of a heart-healthy diet."

You don't need diabetes to benefit from eating the "smiling pistachio" as it's known in Iran. Try to include at least a handful of unsalted pistachios in your diet every day to make yourself — and your heart — smile.

Hit the hay to sleep high blood pressure away. Spending too much time counting sheep? You're missing out on a good opportunity to get your ticker on track. That's because sleep helps regulate your blood pressure.

"Blood flow to your organs is going to change when you are sleeping," says Dr. Daniel Rudic, vascular biologist at the Medical College of Georgia. "Your heart rate is going to decrease."

Rudic explains that blood pressure has a circadian rhythm that matches your sleep-wake cycle. Poor sleep habits will throw it off, and your blood pressure won't drop as it should.

Luckily, you can follow these tips from the latest sleep research.

> If your sleep is disrupted by shift work or sleep apnea, a low-salt diet won't bring your blood pressure down and may even have the opposite effect, a new study shows. Talk to your doctor about ways to build a better night's sleep.

- ▶ **Aim for eight hours of Zzzs.** People who get at least eight hours of sleep each night are more likely to have good heart health than those who get less sleep, studies say.

- ▶ **If you have sleep apnea, get it treated.** Studies show that CPAP therapy or mandibular devices help lower systolic and diastolic blood pressure.

- ▶ **Take a nap.** Out of nearly 400 middle-aged folks with high blood pressure, those who took an hour-long siesta at noon saw their systolic blood pressure reading drop about 5 percent throughout the day.

▸ **Shift your med schedule.** Getting irregular sleep from shift work can affect your pressure and raise your risk for heart disease. While you can't always control your work hours, you may gain better control of your blood pressure by changing the time you take your medication. Talk to your doctor about what time of day will make it most effective.

Groundbreaking treatments lower BP for good

New!

This just in — blood pressure breakthroughs bring your numbers down like never before. These emerging treatments have scientists practically jumping for joy.

Sound therapy. This new tech uses sensors to measure brain electrical activity and detect imbalances that lead to high blood pressure. It turns these frequencies into audible tones that you hear via earbuds. Amazingly, they found it helps balance blood pressure.

Ultrasound. In just 20 minutes, the device lowered systolic BP up to 23 mmHg in diabetes patients with treatment-resistant high blood pressure. Researchers think it calms down the sympathetic nervous system, which is involved in making your heart beat faster, constricting blood vessels, and raising blood pressure.

Modern medicine. A new drug targets nerve signals in the carotid bodies located in arteries that run alongside the neck. This reduces hyperactivity that causes blood pressure to rise. Scientists think this treatment may work better than existing drugs because it controls blood pressure where it commonly starts.

Raise your glass to heart-healing antioxidants. Drink eight 8-ounce glasses of water a day, goes the popular advice. That's because dehydration throws your whole body out of whack, including your blood pressure, which can either plummet or skyrocket. Here's why.

Water pumps up the volume of your blood, helping it to flow more smoothly. When you're dehydrated, there's less pressure against your artery walls, so your blood pressure may drop dangerously low.

On the other hand, your body can react by holding on to sodium to try and increase fluids. That leads to a shutdown of tiny blood vessels called capillaries, increasing the force of blood on your arteries and raising your pressure.

Either way, the key to keeping your blood pressure balanced is to stay hydrated. You don't have to stick to water, but don't turn to sodas and sugary sports drinks. Instead, stock up on antioxidant-packed juices that go the extra mile.

▶ **Cranberry.** This tart drink may get its heart benefits from quercetin, an antioxidant known for lowering blood pressure. It takes about a cup of low-calorie cranberry juice twice a day, according to one study. After eight weeks, diastolic blood pressure in the treatment group dropped an average of 4.7 mmHg and was lower than the placebo group's.

Researchers say that type of change is similar to what you'd get from the heart-friendly DASH diet or a low-sodium diet. The really good news? It may lower your risk of heart disease by 10 percent and your risk of stroke by 15 percent.

▶ **Pomegranate.** This super juice is packed with antioxidants called flavonoids. Drinking just half a cup three times every week for a year reduced blood pressure in patients at high risk for heart disease, says a study published in *Nutrition Journal*.

▶ **Chokeberry.** You may not have heard of chokeberries also called aronia berries — but they are super-rich in polyphenols, a group of potent antioxidants. In a small study, volunteers drank almost a cup of chokeberry juice every day for four weeks. They saw a drop in both systolic and diastolic blood pressure. Look for chokeberry juice in specialty grocery stores or online.

Cut your risk with a creamy favorite. You can freeze it, drink it, or jazz it up with fruit and granola. But yogurt isn't just a yummy treat. It's also a healthy one and is especially kind to your heart, scientists say.

While examining data from two long-term Nurses' Health Studies, researchers noticed a trend in women who ate five or more servings of yogurt each week. They had a 20 percent lower risk of developing high blood pressure compared to those who rarely ate the creamy treat.

"No one food is a magic bullet," says lead author Justin Buendia from Boston University School of Medicine. "But adding yogurt to an otherwise healthy diet seems to help reduce the long-term risk of high blood pressure in women."

In fact, the benefits rose when they ate more fruits, vegetables, nuts, beans, low-fat dairy, and whole grains — signatures of the DASH diet, an eating plan that lowers blood pressure.

Scientists aren't sure why yogurt helps, but previous studies have suggested the bacteria in yogurt may lower cholesterol, which helps keep your arteries clear. And adding yogurt to a wholesome diet can help you maintain a healthy weight, also a boon to your blood pressure.

Not all research agrees with this study, which was funded by the National Dairy Council, so the jury is still out. But it doesn't hurt to stock up your fridge with this tasty treat, and enjoy it regularly.

Tame tension to heal your heart. Some people think the word hypertension means you have too much stress. But it actually has nothing to do with emotional stress. Tension refers to the physical pressure of blood against your artery walls, and hyper means it's way too high.

Maybe this confusion is why less than half of people with high blood pressure have it under control. Lowering blood pressure takes more than just managing your stress levels. That said, adding stress-lowering strategies to your daily routine may be a helpful addition to your other treatments. Try these research-supported ways for relaxing.

- **Tune in to the classics.** Want to rewind high blood pressure? Lay back and listen to Mozart's Symphony No. 40 in G minor. Classical music lowers your blood pressure better than upbeat pop songs like the works of ABBA, a study found. "Dancing Queen" is great for having a ball, but if you want to relax, sit with the symphonies for about 25 minutes.

- **Bring back an ancient practice.** Tai Chi, a gentle, graceful form of exercise, is great for all ages. This Chinese tradition gets its heart-healing powers from fluid movements that focus on posture, coordination, and breathing patterns.

One study showed it lowered systolic blood pressure by more than nine points.

▶ **Simmer down.** By watching married couples have tense conversations for just 15 minutes, researchers could predict who would have health problems more than 20 years later. Are you a hothead? You may be setting yourself up for high blood pressure. Before you lose your temper, take a few deep breaths and calm yourself down.

Open up arteries one sweet treat at a time. Looking for an excuse to slip more chocolate into your week? You don't have to.

Cacao flavanols found in chocolate are powerful antioxidants that are a boon to blood flow, says a study published in the *British Journal of Nutrition*.

Lower blood pressure, heart disease, and diabetes and even reverse memory loss in seniors. Powerful nutrients in natural cocoa can do it all. But don't grab a glass of milk to wash down your dark chocolate treat. Milk can ruin the benefits by keeping antioxidants from being absorbed.

Drinking a flavanol-filled beverage twice a day for a month not only made arteries more open and flexible, it actually lowered systolic blood pressure by 4.4 mmHg and diastolic blood pressure by 3.9 mmHg.

The volunteers were healthy, middle-aged people with no signs of heart disease. So it's never too early to start protecting your heart — and cocoa is a delicious way to do it.

Cocoa powder has the highest amount of flavanols. If you're more of a fan of the chocolate bar, you can follow these tips and still claim the health perks.

- **Go over to the dark side.** You'll get the best benefits from dark chocolate. Avoid added fats and calories from caramel, nougat, and fudge.

- **Don't go overboard.** Cacao is combined with sugar and cocoa butter to make dark chocolate, so aim for less than 1.5 ounces a day.

- **Look over the label.** Search for bars with higher percentages of cacao, which means more flavanols and less sugar.

Relax arteries and boost blood flow with this 'NO' brainer

Beets are one food you probably never think of when writing up your grocery list. But you should, especially if you have high blood pressure.

This crimson vegetable is rich in nitrates, which your body turns into nitric oxide (NO). And nitric oxide is a superstar when it comes to relaxing blood vessels and improving blood flow. Who knew a simple beet could do so much to help your heart?

Why you hear bad things about nitrates. Nitrates are often added to processed foods like bacon and hot dogs to preserve color and keep harmful bacteria from growing. And adding nitrates or nitrites to food can lead to the formation of nitrosamines, which can eventually cause cancer. But nitrates are not harmful when they occur naturally in food because vitamin C in fruits and veggies prevents nitrosamines from forming. Instead, they create nitric oxide, which is beneficial to your body.

Beet juice is a winner when it comes to blood pressure.
Drinking beet juice every day could lower your systolic blood pressure by five to 10 points, says a recent study — even in older people who are already experiencing heart troubles. Other research found similar results. In fact, a British study was the first to show that nitrates in your diet can help lower blood pressure, even if you already have high blood pressure.

> It aids your immune system. It boosts brain power. And when it comes to blood flow, its ability to open up arteries blows the competition away. No wonder nitric oxide was named "molecule of the year" back in 1992.

Researchers divided up 68 volunteers ages 18 to 85 and asked half of them to drink about a cup of beetroot juice every day for a month. The juice helped relax stiff arteries and lowered blood pressure by about 8/4 mmHg. Those in the nitrate-free group did not see any benefits. The best part? Many of the people who were having trouble lowering their blood pressure with drugs saw their pressure drop into the normal range.

Added benefits strengthen beet's appeal. Not only does the nitrate in beets lower your blood pressure, it can also help increase blood flow and oxygen delivery to essential organs and tissues, such as your brain and muscles. As a result, it can raise your energy level, reduce muscle fatigue, and even improve problem-solving skills. Not bad for a vegetable root.

Why you need olive oil on your spinach salad

Who knew?

The tin man from The Wizard of Oz doesn't have a heart. But if he did — and he was smart — he'd make sure his oil can was filled with heart-healthy olive oil. This oil is bursting with polyphenols that can actually lubricate your blood vessels, keeping artery walls smooth and your blood flowing freely.

Pour a little of that olive oil on leafy greens like spinach and arugula, and you'll boost their power to lower your blood pressure, says a study led by King's College London.

Leafy greens are packed with artery-healing nitrates. The combination of unsaturated fats and nitrates creates nitro fatty acids that stop enzymes from hiking your blood pressure.

"This helps explain why previous research has shown that a Mediterranean diet supplemented with extra-virgin olive oil or nuts can reduce cardiovascular problems like stroke, heart failure, and heart attacks," says researcher Philip Eaton.

Fill your plate with heart-healthy choices. You can kick-start your heart health by taking advantage of this natural way to control your blood pressure. Not crazy about beets? Try other high-nitrate foods like arugula, spinach, Swiss chard, fennel, beet greens, basil, spring greens, cilantro, and rhubarb.

Do It Better

BP mistakes that sabotage your readings (and how to fix them)

Have you ever stopped by the gym or sipped a cup of coffee on the way to your doctor appointment? Those things can temporarily raise your blood pressure and change your reading. Put these tips into practice to improve accuracy up to 50 points.

Cuff correctly. Using a tight cuff or placing it over your wooly sweater could hike blood pressure results.

Measure again. Anxiety, or the "white coat" effect, can spike blood pressure. Measure again at the end of your appointment when you're more relaxed.

Match monitors. Home monitors can be inaccurate, especially apps that don't have cuffs. Take yours to your appointment to compare with your doctor's.

Relieve yourself. That "gotta go" feeling does more than ruin a good movie. A full bladder can also raise blood pressure.

Perfect posture. Sit quietly with your feet flat on the floor, and make sure your arm is supported at heart level.

DASH diet update: how to get even more powerful results

The DASH diet is the go-to plan if you want to successfully lower your blood pressure. It stands for Dietary Approaches to Stop Hypertension, and it can help bring down your blood pressure in just 14 days. What's more, it may lower cholesterol and fight heart disease, stroke, kidney disease, and some cancers.

As good as it is, new research shows you can tweak the eating plan to make it work even better. How? Make it entirely plant-based. Although vegetables, fruits, and whole grains are the heart of the DASH diet, the plan also allows you to eat meats, poultry, and fish.

Scientists have always known that people who eat plant-based diets have lower blood pressure and risk of stroke. So when they created the DASH diet, they wanted it to offer similar benefits. So why isn't DASH vegetarian? Well, the group in charge decided the eating plan had to appeal to the average American. They reasoned that people wouldn't stick to a diet that didn't include at least some meat.

But studies say, when it comes to lowering blood pressure, the more plants the better. In fact, one study looked at blood pressure data from 500 people enrolled in the long-term Adventist Health Study-2. Researchers found a significant difference between the meat-and-vegetable eaters and those who ate a meatless diet of fruits, veggies, and low-fat dairy. The average systolic blood pressure in the meatless group was about nine points lower. Diastolic pressure was almost six points lower.

Now the secret is out. You can take your heart-healthy DASH meal plan to the next level by cutting out meat and piling on the veggies.

Shake the habit — salt substitutes that can save your heart

Forty-four thousand. That's the number of Americans who could be saved each year by merely eating less salt — just a half teaspoon less per day. It's really not as surprising as it sounds. This mineral is a bad guy when it comes to blood pressure, and it's not so good for the rest of you either.

Bad news for your body. Salt is made up of two elements — sodium and chloride. Sodium pulls water into your bloodstream, increasing the volume of blood zooming through your body. This extra fluid makes your heart pump harder, raising your blood pressure and damaging your arteries.

Try this trick from dietitian Jeff Novick. Don't buy foods that have more milligrams (mg) of sodium than calories. Say you're the average Joe eating about 2,000 calories a day. If everything you munch on has less sodium than calories, you'll meet the American Heart Association's suggestion of less than 2,300 mg.

But that's not all you have to worry about. If your blood pressure is fine, you may think you can munch on all the salty snacks you want. Not so fast. Even if you don't have high blood pressure, extra salt can damage other organs, hiking up your risk of heart disease, kidney disease, and stroke.

Sneaky ways sodium gets into your diet. Maybe you're patting yourself on the back for leaving the saltshaker on the table. That's a good start, but it's only a small part of the problem.

"About 70 percent of the sodium in our diets comes from processed foods, including items that we don't typically think of as salty, such as breads and cereals," says William Weintraub, chief of cardiology at Christiana Care Health System. "Also, restaurant food typically contains more salt than dishes prepared at home, so eating out less can help reduce salt intake, especially if herbs and spices — instead of salt — are used to add flavor to home-cooked meals."

Sub out salt with flavorful stand-ins. You can find many creative ways to cut down on salt in the kitchen. One of the most popular options is garlic. This powerful herb can lower blood pressure, regulate cholesterol, and stimulate your immune system. How? Antioxidant activity. That's how it helps prevent the top three killer ailments — heart disease, cancer, and stroke.

Don't forget about these tasty, heart-healing spices that have been around for years.

- parsley
- onion
- cinnamon

- ginseng
- ginger
- saffron

- cilantro
- sweet basil
- cardamom

Warning

Recipe for disaster — skip ingredients that bump up BP

You know the old saying "you are what you eat." But what about "you are *when* you eat"? It's true. When you eat could have a big effect on your blood pressure. Ted didn't know it either until his doctor told him his high blood pressure may be linked to skipping meals and eating later in the day.

Of course, *what* you eat can harm you too. That's why Ted's doctor advised him to stay away from these pressure-boosting ingredients.

Caffeine. If you're big on coffee and energy drinks, watch out. Not only are they high in caffeine, both drinks contain other compounds and stimulants that may raise your BP.

Alcohol. Drinking too much can sabotage your blood pressure. Experts suggest low-alcohol or nonalcoholic varieties.

Sugar. Fructose is the offender in many sodas and fruit drinks. One study found your blood pressure could jump 1.6 mmHg for every extra sugar-sweetened beverage you drink each day.

High cholesterol

Have you ever tried drinking a thick milkshake through a straw? The ice cream clogs up the narrow passageway, making it almost impossible to enjoy. That's what happens to your arteries when they're overloaded with cholesterol. But instead of brain freeze, you could face a more serious threat.

The good, the bad, and the ugly side of cholesterol. Cholesterol gets a bad rap because of its association with heart disease. But it's not like this waxy substance hangs around your arteries waiting to plug them up and give you a heart attack. Cholesterol actually has important jobs to do in your body, such as making hormones, vitamin D, and bile.

The problem is that too much of it can create a traffic jam in your arteries. The excess cholesterol attaches itself to the artery wall, along with other substances like fat and calcium. These all harden into a substance called plaque, which narrows the opening your blood flows through. This road block can cut off blood and oxygen to your heart or brain, leading to a heart attack or stroke.

Carriers shepherd cholesterol to and fro. Cholesterol doesn't wander through your arteries on its own. Small particles called lipoproteins act as carriers to escort cholesterol to its proper destination. Low-density lipoproteins (LDL) are notoriously referred to as "bad" cholesterol because those are the ones that stick around and create a plaque pileup in your arteries.

High-density lipoproteins (HDL), on the other hand, absorb and taxi cholesterol to the liver, where it's flushed from the body. High levels of HDL can slash your risk for heart problems, which is why people often call it "good" cholesterol.

High levels often start in the kitchen. Your body makes all the cholesterol it needs, so for most people, food is their downfall. But it's not high-cholesterol foods like eggs and shrimp that cause the problem. New research shows foods high in cholesterol don't have as big of an impact as people once thought.

Instead, saturated fat and trans fat are the culprits. Dietitians recommend you steer clear of trans fat and eat less saturated fat, because they can cause your LDL levels to skyrocket. That means you need to take it easy on the steak and buttery biscuits.

Check out your numbers regularly. High cholesterol has no symptoms, so the only way you'll know you have a problem is through testing. Doctors say everyone over age 20 should get their cholesterol levels checked at least once every five years.

Aim for a total cholesterol score of less than 200 milligrams per deciliter (mg/dL). This score includes LDL, HDL, and triglycerides, which are fats that can contribute to gridlock in your arteries.

Although cholesterol levels are heavily influenced by factors you can't control, such as age, heredity, and gender, you do have control over some things. Your food choices are one of them. Here are some foods you should be eating regularly, especially if you're over 55 years old. They'll help clean and flush out your arteries.

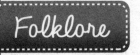

'Good' cholesterol may not be as good as you think

It's one of the first things you learn about cholesterol — HDL is good for you, and the more you have the better. So you may think your cholesterol is fine as long as your HDL levels are skyrocketing. Turns out, new research says it doesn't work that way.

LDL and HDL are not as black and white as you think, and focusing on just one type could put your heart in jeopardy. High HDL cholesterol is linked to a 20-to-40-percent lower risk for heart disease. But this benefit may be canceled out when LDL and triglyceride levels are 100 mg/dL or higher.

Make sure you focus on an overall healthy diet and lifestyle because high HDL levels alone are not enough to protect you from heart disease.

15 foods that clean your arteries

Give your arteries a good scrub naturally with broccoli. You used to sneak those little green trees under the table to Fido, but now you may want to hang onto your broccoli. Recent research shows these veggies may help slow havoc caused by atherosclerosis, the hardening and narrowing of blood vessels. Even better — broccoli may help reverse the damage.

Broccoli and other cruciferous vegetables, such as Brussels sprouts and cabbage, contain sulforaphane. This nutrient may turn back the clock on heart damage by boosting enzymes that fight off oxidative stress and inflammation.

In a recent study out of Egypt, sulforaphane lowered "bad" cholesterol while boosting "good" cholesterol and improving blood flow. Although the researchers tested sulforaphane supplements on animals, they suggest people with high cholesterol could benefit by including more of these vegetables in their diet.

'No fasting' rule makes test — and your life — easier

New!

Wouldn't it be nice if you could test your cholesterol without having to fast? That rumbly in your tumbly, as Pooh Bear would say, may be a thing of the past. New research out of Europe shows the test may be just as accurate when you don't go on a hunger strike beforehand.

The study, published in *European Heart Journal*, made an international recommendation that fasting is no longer necessary before cholesterol and triglyceride testing. Their research shows cholesterol and triglyceride levels don't change much whether you eat something ahead of time or not.

Talk to your doctor at your next visit to see if you can take advantage of this proposed rule.

Go nuts to control your cholesterol. When you hear the words "tree nuts," you might think of squirrels hiding away acorns for the winter. Actually, tree nuts include crowd favorites such as almonds, cashews, pecans, pistachios, walnuts, Brazil nuts, and more.

These nutty nibbles are great for your ticker. A recent study published in *Nutrition Journal* shows that eating about one-quarter cup of tree nuts each day can help you lose pounds, cut blood pressure, and raise HDL levels — the "good" cholesterol. They also have a history of lowering LDL cholesterol and triglycerides, both of which can contribute to heart disease.

Walnuts have a particularly good rep. Researchers found that total and LDL cholesterol levels drop when people eat walnuts every day. These nuts are packed with nutrients such as folate, B vitamins, magnesium, and good fats.

So feel free to add a handful to your morning breakfast or snack. It's one easy thing you can do every day to lower your cholesterol.

Crunch more fiber to take a bite out of "bad" cholesterol.
Barley just may be the new No. 1 food for reducing your cholesterol. And its extra fiber comes with splendid side effects — a slimmer waist, lower blood pressure, and smaller risk for diabetes.

Oats have long been the go-to grain for heart health. Their golden ingredient — a soluble fiber known as beta-glucan — has even won the approval of the U.S. Food and Drug Administration (FDA). The FDA allows food labels to boast that their whole-oat products lower cholesterol if they provide 3 or more grams of beta-glucan daily.

Recently, barley was also added to the claim. The latest studies show that barley, a rich source of beta-glucan, has similar cholesterol-lowering effects. And a cup of barley boasts four times the amount of fiber and double the protein of a cup of oatmeal.

Researchers analyzed 14 studies in which participants ate about 7 grams of beta-glucan every day. That would equal a little under three cups of cooked barley. After four weeks, their LDL cholesterol dropped. And yours can too.

If you eat just one thing for breakfast, make it this superfood. You can add cinnamon and fruit for a tasty start to your day. And try it out on salad, in soup, and as a substitute for rice in recipes like risotto.

Try this sweet way to raise good cholesterol. Brown fuzzy peel and bright green pulp — kiwifruit sure does know how to make an impression.

And that's not the only thing it's good for. A recent study published in *Nutrition Journal* shows that people who eat one or more kiwi each week have higher HDL "good" cholesterol and lower triglycerides than those who leave them at the supermarket.

This isn't the first study to hint at the cholesterol-improving effects of kiwi. Scientists think their healing powers come from polyphenols and vitamin C. These nutrients help lower blood fats and strengthen your blood vessels, which lowers your risk of heart disease.

Experts say you should get 75 to 90 milligrams of vitamin C daily. Snack on one of these sweet fruits a day to get on the right track.

Protect your arteries with a yummy combo. A pomegranate tree could live to be 200 years old. While it won't help you live that long, the ruby-red fruit is packed with antioxidants that may help your heart beat longer.

Small studies continue to show pomegranate juice helps reduce blood pressure, cholesterol, and inflammation. In one surprising study published in an Israeli medical journal, the tasty juice helped certain statins shield cells from oxidative stress.

Looking for a new way to enjoy this cholesterol-demolishing juice? In a recent animal study, a pomegranate juice and date cocktail lowered LDL cholesterol and triglyceride levels. This delicious duo safeguards against plaque buildup and hardened arteries, which can cause a heart attack or stroke. The protection is mostly due to polyphenols, plant nutrients that act as antioxidants. They are known for striking back at cancer, diabetes, stroke, and heart disease.

The researchers say you'll get the most artery protection from eating three dates with their pits along with half a glass of pomegranate juice each day. But if you're not up to grinding date pits, you'll still benefit from just the date-juice combination. Try blending the two with your favorite fruits in a smoothie.

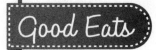 **Easy trick makes eating pomegranates a snap**

The pomegranate has hundreds of tiny juice sacs held together by a leathery skin. These "seeds" are great in salads and other dishes or eaten alone as a healthy snack. The trick is to separate the tasty juice from the rest of the fruit, which is tough and bitter.

An easy way is to cut the fruit into pieces and put them into a bowl of water, then scoop the tiny sacs out with your fingers. When you're done, remove the skin, strain out the water, and enjoy the luscious fruit that's left.

Clear up clogs with a heart-y seed. What if you could cut your cholesterol by eating muffins, bagels, pasta, and cereal? Sounds good, doesn't it? As long as those foods contained flaxseed, you'd be on the right track.

That's what Canadian researchers found during a yearlong study of volunteers with peripheral artery disease, a sign of clogged arteries. The volunteers ate foods like these containing 30 grams (g) — about 2 tablespoons — of ground flaxseed every day. After just one month, their LDL cholesterol had dropped by 15 percent and their total cholesterol by 11 percent.

Another study showed that taking 3 g of flaxseed oil a day, in addition to following a healthy diet, lowered LDL and total cholesterol in 12 weeks. Even better — the flax oil also raised HDL levels significantly.

These tiny seeds are jam-packed with nutrients, including soluble fiber, lignans, and alpha-linolenic acid, an essential fatty acid. It's possible one or more of these contribute to their cholesterol-lowering abilities. Start getting the benefits today by adding flaxseed to baked goods, smoothies, yogurt, and more. Or sprinkle some flax oil on your favorite salad.

One easy way to keep the heart doctor away. A lot of health advice has fallen out of favor in the face of scientific findings, but "an apple a day" keeps proving itself again and again.

Research reveals this fruit not only lowers cholesterol but is also a heart-attack stopper. And, amazingly, it may work as well as medication.

▶ Postmenopausal women who ate dried apples every day for a year saw a 23 percent drop in bad LDL cholesterol, along with a 4 percent rise in HDL cholesterol, says a study out of Florida State University. Researchers think the pectin and polyphenols in apples help clear cholesterol from the blood and protect against inflammation.

▶ British researchers compared apples to statin drugs to determine how well they each protected against heart attack, stroke, and other vascular problems. They were surprised to learn the apples performed almost as well as the statins. They estimate that by snacking on apples every day, people could avoid or delay 8,500 heart attacks and strokes each year — and help stave off diabetes.

Chalk another one up for grandma's home remedies.

Rx Alert

Statin side effect: diabetes risk is real

Statins are some of the most prescribed drugs in America. With more than 20 million annual prescriptions of Crestor alone, it's likely you or someone you know is taking a cholesterol-lowering drug. Statins can be life changing, but make sure you get all the information before you take them. These powerful pills come with a serious potential side effect.

The latest news, from a study of more than 8,000 men, shows statin treatment can hike the risk of type 2 diabetes by 46 percent. Researchers say it's because they could cause drops in insulin sensitivity and secretion.

The Food and Drug Administration has recognized this increased risk, but they say statins' benefits for preventing heart disease may outweigh the risk. Be sure to talk to your health care provider, so you understand how the drug may affect you.

Spice keeps harmful fats from heaping up. Turmeric is one of the latest health-food darlings. You may not recognize the spice, but you've eaten it before, whether you realize it or not.

Turmeric is found in mustard, curry, cheeses, and butters. It has a powerful ingredient called curcumin, which gives these foods their staple yellow color. But it also does much more than that, especially for your arteries.

Curcumin helps scavenger cells, called macrophages, remove harmful fats from your body, and also lessens inflammation. That helps keep your blood vessels smooth and plaque-free. Plus, it slashes LDL cholesterol and triglycerides — a type of blood fat — while raising HDL levels.

Every little bit helps when it comes to controlling cholesterol. Adding a little turmeric to your stir-fries, soups, vegetables, even scrambled eggs, may give your arteries just the healthy boost they need.

Tackle high cholesterol with (surprise) high-fat avocados. Here's something you may not know — avocados are actually berries. And that's not the only surprise they have in store. Despite being high in fat, they are a valuable weapon in the fight against heart disease.

These "berries" are rich in monounsaturated fatty acids (MUFAs), which help bring down cholesterol and triglyceride levels. But it's not just the fatty acids that give heart disease the heave-ho. Avocados are also rich in heart-healthy fiber, vitamins, minerals, polyphenols, and phytosterols.

Adding a daily avocado to a moderate-fat diet helps lower your cholesterol better than eating a low- or moderate-fat diet, even if they're high in MUFAs, researchers found. They believe the extra nutrients in avocados make the difference.

If you'd like to enjoy more avocados, make sure you cut back on other high-fat foods. Here's one yummy idea — ditch the butter and mayo, and make an avocado spread for your toast and sandwiches.

Coffee delivers a one-two punch. Mmm, that morning cup of coffee is just what you need to get your blood flowing. Literally.

A recent study showed that coffee helps prevent calcium buildup in the arteries of your heart — an early sign of heart disease. That buildup, called calcification, leads to artery-clogging plaque, which limits blood flow to your heart.

Out of 25,000 people studied by South Korean scientists, those who drank between three and five cups of joe each day showed the lowest levels of calcification. Researchers think several factors may be responsible for coffee's positive effects. But previous studies have shown mixed results about coffee and heart health, so more research is needed.

Before you turn your kitchen into a barista haven, keep in mind you need to drink filtered coffee. The study points out that unfiltered coffee, like French press or Turkish, raises your cholesterol. And high cholesterol plays a big role in heart disease.

Get rid of bad cholesterol with good bacteria. For life. That's the meaning of the word probiotic — an appropriate name for the good bacteria that keep your gut — and your health — in balance.

Researchers studying weight loss wanted to know whether these special bacteria could help people shed pounds. For 12 weeks, volunteers ate either probiotic yogurt or low-fat yogurt with their main meals while following a weight-loss program. The probiotics didn't seem to affect weight, but they produced a significant drop in LDL and total cholesterol. The probiotic group also had better blood levels of fat and insulin.

To get these benefits from yogurt, make sure you choose one packed with probiotics. Look for a label that says "contains live and active cultures" or has the name of specific bacteria in the ingredients list. One study suggests *Lactobacillus acidophilus* strains lower LDL best.

Break up plaque buildup with garlic. Garlic may not be the sweetest smelling remedy, but dozens of early studies show that allium, a phytochemical found in garlic, can help lower cholesterol. Other studies say garlic doesn't have remarkable effects. So what's the latest news?

The most recent research from the *Journal of Nutrition* supports the heart-healthy benefits of garlic.

▶ A review of research on garlic supplementation shows garlic lowers total cholesterol by about 7 to 30 mg/dL.

▶ Another study revealed 2,400 milligrams of aged garlic extract daily can lower dangerous plaque buildup in a way similar to statin therapy.

Some studies have used supplements, some powdered garlic, and some raw garlic. It's up to you. For a simple solution, slip a couple cloves of garlic into your menu each day.

Is black garlic the new superfood?

New!

Aged black garlic is the new novelty ingredient of top chefs around the world. Rumor is, this delicious delicacy is tender and doesn't leave you with bad breath. But is it healthier than fresh garlic?

Ferment garlic for several weeks with special equipment, and the result is a black bulb that's not pungent like the garlic you're used to. Black garlic does have strong antioxidant properties, and one animal study showed that it may help control cholesterol. But in another study, aged garlic did not fight inflammation as well as fresh garlic, which is cheaper and easier to find.

Human studies are limited, and not all scientists agree that black garlic is the new superfood. Feel free to try it fresh or as a supplement, but don't expect it to revolutionize your health.

Go cuckoo for cocoa to cut down cholesterol. Want another great reason to eat chocolate? Cocoa beans might help you lower LDL cholesterol in just one month.

In recent studies, cocoa extract also raised HDL cholesterol, the good kind that helps remove extra fats from your blood and prevent plaque buildup. Researchers think this benefit comes from flavanols found in foods such as grapes, apples, tea, and of course, chocolate.

You can slip cocoa into your diet to reap the heart-healthy benefits of these flavanols. But think twice before you load up on your favorite chocolate bars. They're usually loaded with calories, fat, and sugar.

It's best to choose dark chocolate over milk chocolate and aim for a high percentage of cocoa or cacao. When you shop for cocoa powder, look for one that is made without Dutch processing, a technique that destroys flavanols.

Trick your gut with an LDL look-alike. Phytosterols are masters of disguise. They look so similar to cholesterol that your gut often absorbs them instead of the bad guys. That results in lower levels of cholesterol in your blood.

So what are phytosterols? They're compounds found in all plant foods such as fruits, vegetables, nuts, seeds, grain products, and vegetable oils. Studies have found that 3 grams of phytosterols a day can lower LDL cholesterol by about 12 percent. The problem is that most plants only contain small amounts. You'd need to eat a cup of sesame seeds to get just over 1 gram of sterols. That's a lot even for your favorite stir-fry.

Luckily, you have another option — fortified foods. The FDA recognizes sterols' health benefits and encourages people to include sterol-fortified foods in their diet. Margarine is one popular source. Look for products like Benecol and Take Control in your local supermarket. You'll also find sterol-fortified orange juice, granola bars, cheeses, chocolates, and cooking oils. Just keep an eye on the calories and fats in the products you choose.

Sterols don't interfere with cholesterol-lowering drugs like statins, so you don't have to worry about interactions. Studies show they actually work together to provide a one-two punch against high cholesterol.

Ketchup's secret weapon battles free radicals. This saucy condiment is good for more than just flavoring your burger and fries. Research proves that lycopene, found naturally in tomatoes and tomato-based products like ketchup, may help lower your cholesterol naturally.

Lycopene is an antioxidant that wipes out free radicals before they can attach to cells and cause problems such as inflammation. When LDL cholesterol meets up with free radicals it becomes damaged — or oxidized — and eventually turns into plaque that clogs up your arteries.

One study showed that tomato juice, spaghetti sauce, and concentrated lycopene all helped double blood levels of lycopene and significantly lower oxidized LDL. And, amazingly, they did the job in just one week.

In analyzing more than 55 years of lycopene studies, scientists found this super antioxidant drops LDL levels by about 10 percent, similar to low doses of statin drugs. Study participants ate at least 25 milligrams of lycopene each day — the amount found in a cup of tomato juice or less than half a cup of spaghetti sauce.

Those foods are easy to add to your daily menu, and they're healthier than a ketchup-laden burger and fries. Here are some other ways to add lycopene to your meals.

▶ Breakfast — eat half a pink grapefruit.

▶ Lunch — enjoy a warm bowl of tomato soup.

▶ Dinner — dig into a hearty meal of pasta and marinara sauce. Or enjoy a low-cheese pizza with sun-dried tomatoes and plenty of sauce.

▶ Dessert — have a slice of watermelon.

Is high cholesterol robbing you of vitamin E?

Sure, your doctor warns you about the dangers of high cholesterol, but you can worry about that later, right? What if he told you all that cholesterol in your bloodstream is weakening your immune system right now?

A study published in the *American Journal of Clinical Nutrition* says high cholesterol may interfere with your body's ability to absorb vitamin E, a powerful immune-system booster. This critical fat-soluble antioxidant helps protect your body against cell-damaging free radicals and inflammation. It also prevents LDL from oxidizing, which contributes to heart disease.

High levels of cholesterol and triglycerides keep vitamin E circulating in your bloodstream, which means it's not getting absorbed into tissues that need the immunity boost. So make sure you follow your doctor's advice on lowering your cholesterol. And try to get at least 15 milligrams of vitamin E every day by eating foods like nuts, whole grains, leafy greens, and vegetable oils.

Beat high cholesterol with a slower lifestyle

"For fast-acting relief, try slowing down," quips comedian Lily Tomlin. It's great advice for a number of health woes, high cholesterol included.

A stressful life causes changes in your bloodstream. It spikes fats like triglycerides and can also raise the level of chemicals called cytokines that promote inflammation. Research has shown that stress is associated with inflammation, hardened arteries, and high cholesterol.

▸ Police officers under high stress had higher levels of triglycerides, lower levels of HDL cholesterol, and a greater risk of developing metabolic syndrome, one study showed.

▸ Job stress was linked to high "bad" LDL cholesterol and low "good" HDL cholesterol in a study involving more than 90,000 people. In fact, researchers say being stressed increases your chances of a high cholesterol diagnosis.

When things get tough, pick your favorite stress release, like listening to music or sipping chamomile tea, and give yourself a chance to relax. But don't forget the things you can do every day to keep your stress levels — and your cholesterol — in check.

Shut down plaque pileup with a bit of shuteye. Missing a good night's sleep throws off a lot of things in your body, and cholesterol is one of them. Studies show sleep loss can crank up inflammation and triglycerides as well as lower HDL cholesterol. This bumps up your risk for heart problems.

Even throwing off your regular sleep schedule can have heart consequences. Waking early on workdays and sleeping in on weekends is known as social jet lag. A recent study shows this type of lifestyle can lower HDL and raise triglycerides. It's also linked to diabetes and hardening and narrowing of the arteries. So try to be consistent and catch enough sleep each night.

Get moving to lower stress — and protect your heart. Exercise doesn't just burn off stress. People who get moving have better

HDL cholesterol and triglyceride levels and a lower risk of heart disease. Here's what studies have to say.

▸ Every extra minute spent being a couch potato could lead to a dip in your good cholesterol — a 0.03 mg/dL drop among folks with heart disease and 0.02 mg/dL in those without heart troubles.

▸ Each extra hour of time spent sitting around is linked to a 12 percent higher chance of calcium buildup in your arteries. This pileup increases your odds of heart problems.

▸ Being active has long-term effects, too. In a study of more than 11,000 men, those who were physically fit kept healthy cholesterol levels 15 years longer than those who weren't.

So add a little more movement to your day. Stand up and do squats or arm lifts during TV commercials, take a walk outside with your pooch, or invite your grandkids over for a dance party.

Worried about weight gain? Don't ditch mealtime. It's no surprise that being overweight is associated with heart disease risk. But if you've ever skipped a few meals to kick-start weight loss, you may want to check out the latest studies.

Eating regularly is not only associated with smaller waistlines but also higher HDL cholesterol and lower LDL cholesterol. One reason may be that meal patterns influence the level of fats in your bloodstream, researchers suggest. More research needs to be done, but don't play hooky at the kitchen table unless your doctor gives you a reason.

Laughter is good for the soul — and your heart

Who Knew?

High cholesterol is no laughing matter — but laughing may help your heart by boosting levels of HDL, or good cholesterol.

In a yearlong study of people with type 2 diabetes, high blood pressure, and high cholesterol, those who watched 30 minutes of funny movies or sitcoms each day in addition to their standard treatment reaped the benefits.

After just two months, their HDL levels improved. After four months, they also lowered blood levels of certain inflammatory chemicals associated with heart disease.

Another good reason to enjoy your favorite comedy shows as often as possible.

Motion sickness

Motion sickness can ruin a trip faster than you can say "stop the world, I want to get off." You get that awful sick-to-your-stomach feeling. You break out in a cold sweat, your head starts to pound, and you feel cranky. You may even vomit. What a terrible way to travel.

Motion sickness happens when your brain receives two conflicting messages — that your body is both moving and still.

Say you're riding in a car reading a book. Your inner ear picks up the signal that your body is moving. But your eyes tell your brain you're not moving at all. These mixed messages confuse your brain's balance center, and your body responds violently.

Recognize the symptoms early, and you have a fighting chance. But wait, and your only recourse may be to stop the car and let it pass.

Arm yourself with these tips to stop motion sickness in its tracks.

3 smart strategies take the misery out of motion

Be prepared wherever you go. Whether you're traveling by train, plane, or automobile, motion sickness can kick in when you're on the move.

Car travel is the most common form of transportation, with over 100 million automobiles on U.S. roads. Don't be a queasy rider on your next road trip.

▸ Offer to drive. This keeps your eyes focused on the road ahead and not the moving scenery.

▸ If you must go as a passenger, call "shotgun" and ride in the front seat.

▸ Don't read while the car is in motion.

▸ Roll down the windows to get fresh air or open a vent.

▸ Apply a cold pack to your face.

▸ Always face forward.

▸ Close your eyes to minimize the mixed signals to your brain.

Are you more of a rowboat or a sailboat? Do you prefer a dinghy or a yacht? Doesn't matter, waves can make you go green regardless of your vessel. Find your sea legs with these tips.

▸ Look to the horizon.

▸ Focus on a fixed spot.

▸ Sit in the middle of a small boat.

▸ On a cruise ship, book a cabin with a window or balcony in the center of the ship.

Close to 900 million passengers flew in and out of the U.S. last year. If you're looking to jet away anytime soon, keep the skies friendly.

▸ Turn your air vent on and point it toward your face.

▸ Sit toward the front of the plane or in the middle over the wings.

Digital motion can turn you green

Who Knew?

"Don't ask me to take a seat at a video arcade to race cars or fly planes," says Annie from Atlanta. "Watching all that movement on a screen makes me nauseous in no time flat."

It's called cybersickness — a digital motion sickness prevalent in today's super tech world. The direct opposite of regular motion sickness, it can happen any time your eyes see movement that your body doesn't feel. Your brain's balance center gets mixed messages and the results are headache, dizziness, and nausea.

Even watching an action movie or changing screens rapidly on your smartphone can induce it.

Experts say you can try to overcome cybersickness by engaging in the activity repeatedly. Take breaks when you feel symptoms coming on, then try again.

Women are more susceptible than men and for Annie, it's not worth it. "I'll stick to other games," she says. "I never get sick playing on a pinball machine."

Avoid mistakes that make motion sickness worse. Does the thought of traveling turn your stomach even before you hit the road? Then it's time to address the problem in advance. Here's a list of things you should avoid before and during travel.

▸ Stay away from strong food odors and other scents like perfume.

- Don't eat foods that make you feel full. Stick with light, protein-rich meals or snack on a protein bar.

- Say no to alcohol.

- Steer clear of salty foods, spicy meals, and dairy products.

- Put your cigarettes away if you're a smoker.

Find relief at your corner drugstore. Sometimes the only thing that works comes from your local pharmacy.

Experts say over-the-counter medications like Bonine and Dramamine, and prescriptions like the Transderm Scop patch, all work well. Ask your doctor if one of these is right for you.

But if you want to go drug-free, try acupressure bands that wrap around your wrists. A plastic stud in each band applies pressure to a specific point on your wrist to relieve nausea and vomiting. One reusable pair costs anywhere from $5 to $13, making this a thrifty option.

Ginger: a spicy way to quell your queasies

It's peppery and a little sweet. It's fragrant and it's spicy. It's also gnarly and bumpy. But the root of the ginger plant adds such a special flavor to stir-fries, fruits, and vegetables, no one cares what it looks like. And you'll especially love it if you suffer from motion sickness.

Medicinal ginger goes way back — as in thousands of years back. Ancient cultures in Asia, India, and the Middle East used the herb to treat everything from colds and fever to urinary problems and joint pain. But ginger is perhaps best-known as a remedy against digestive complaints, particularly the nausea that accompanies motion sickness.

It even prevented nausea in clinical studies as well as several motion sickness drugs. Experts think it's the gingerol, a powerful compound in ginger, that thwarts that icky feeling. So make sure you reach for a product with real ginger in it.

Surprisingly, ginger ale may not be your best choice — you'll rarely know how much honest-to-goodness ginger, and not just ginger flavoring, is in a can or a bottle, if any.

You're better off reaching for ginger root powder or capsules, dried ginger slices, or perhaps ginger that's been pickled, crystalized, or even covered in chocolate. While ginger chews and candies may contain the real thing, you should check labels to be sure.

Herbalists believe ginger's spicy fresh scent can also heal churning tummies. Make a simple spritz by combining 12 drops of ginger essential oil with 2 ounces of water in a small, dark bottle. Shake and spray in your car before you hit the road.

Ginger balls

Carry these treats by land, air, or sea for a tasty way to keep motion sickness at bay.

Combine 1 tablespoon of ground ginger, 1 tablespoon of cocoa powder, and 1/2 tablespoon cinnamon.

Mix in enough honey to form a dough. Add a few drops of water to moisten, or more ginger, cocoa, or cinnamon to thicken. Shape into small balls, about the size of a pea.

Make your ginger treats even tastier by rolling them in a bowl of finely chopped nuts or shredded coconut.

Allow them to dry, then store in an airtight container in your fridge for up to a month. Pop in your mouth before or at the onset of motion sickness symptoms.

Muscle cramps

Charley horse. A sweet, gentle name for a sudden, searing pain. You know the signs. It begins with an ominous twinge in the arch of your foot. Before you know it, that twinge swells into an agonizing spasm that grabs hold of your calf and won't let go. For the love of Pete, what, exactly, is going on?

The bad news is, you've got irritated nerves in your stressed muscle that are releasing up to 150 electrical discharges every second, forcing that muscle into a tight squeeze. Ow. No wonder it hurts. The lion's share of cramps — about 90 percent — occur in your thigh, hamstring, or calf.

Experts aren't sure what causes muscle cramps to fire up, but here are some possibilities.

Everyday stress and strain. Your cramps might be the result of overworked muscles in hot weather, sitting too long without moving, or standing too long on hard surfaces. Did you drink enough fluids while working out? If not, dehydration may be the culprit behind your cramps.

Your leg pain's connected to your back pain. The nerves in your lower back may be pinched or compressed because the open spaces within your spine have narrowed, a condition called spinal stenosis. This can cause your legs to cramp. See your doctor for diagnosis and treatment options.

You might be missing minerals. Low levels of calcium, sodium, potassium, or magnesium in your body could be the problem.

Snack on some string cheese to hike up your calcium, chow down on a sweet potato to raise your potassium, and add in some almonds for a magnesium boost.

Check your medications. Prescription drugs can play a part in your discomfort, including:

▶ the calcium channel blocker nifedipine (Procardia).

▶ the Alzheimer's drug donepezil hydrochloride (Aricept).

▶ diuretics like furosemide (Lasix).

▶ some cholesterol-lowering statins.

Talk to your doctor about the side effects of any medicines you're taking.

What are the chances you'll be hobbled by painful muscle cramps? Researchers suspect that age is one contributing factor. You lose muscle mass as you get older, so the muscles get stressed more easily. In a study of 233 people over age 60, almost one-third experienced cramps. For the over-80 crowd it was even worse. Half the people in that age group suffered at least one muscle cramp during the previous two months.

Liver, nerve, or thyroid disorders can cause you to develop cramps. So can diabetes and kidney disease. Obesity also raises your risk.

Do you smoke? Drink lots of coffee? Cut out the nicotine and caffeine, and you'll slash your risk for developing muscle spasms and cramps.

So what should you do the next time you're hit with this middle-of-the-night misery? Here are five home remedies that will bring you sweet relief in a jiffy.

5 fixes for painful cramps

Rub aches away with fragrant massages. Don't let a muscle cramp get a leg up on you. Keep geranium essential oil and evening primrose oil on hand to stop a cramp in progress. First apply 1 teaspoon of evening primrose oil to the affected area. Next rub in 4 drops of geranium essential oil. Continue massaging until the cramp stops. Repeat up to three times a day as needed.

You'll be glad to have this next soothing preparation at your fingertips when your muscles cramp up. Combine four parts of a carrier oil — like olive, coconut, or sweet almond oil — to one part basil essential oil. Massage into your sore muscles. Try taking a hot bath before you apply the oils for more intense results.

Surprising sour power calms your cramps. Sip a little pickle juice, you say? Weird, but true. Researchers studied a group of dehydrated men who were experiencing muscle cramps after exercising. They found those who drank just one-third cup of dill pickle juice got relief from their cramps 37 percent faster than those men who downed the same amount of water.

What gives pickle juice its healing power? Even the experts are baffled, but they suspect the vinegar in the juice may block the nerve signals that make your muscles cramp. In addition, pickle juice contains lots of sodium and even some potassium, the minerals your body needs to recover from a strenuous workout. Just beware. If you're on a low-sodium diet, check with your doctor before you make pickle juice a regular part of your after-exercise routine.

Soak in Epsom salts to soothe your soreness. They're not flashy. They're not fancy. But they work.

Epsom salts are rich in magnesium, a mineral your body needs for healthy muscles. When dissolved in your bath, the magnesium is absorbed though your skin to relax tense muscles, reduce inflammation, and help control electric impulses in your body.

Take three salt baths each week for best results. Simply add two cups of Epsom salts to your warm bath water, and soak for at least 12 minutes. Do not use soap because it will make the salts less effective. Try to rest for about two hours afterward.

A dollop of mustard can wallop your cramps. The spicy spread that makes hot dogs worth eating, and a sandwich sheer delight, is behind an amazing trick to stop leg cramps immediately.

Historians believe the Romans were the first to mix mustard seeds and wine or vinegar to make a paste. Then French monks got in on the act, combining ground mustard seeds with unfermented wine and naming it "mustard," from the Latin for "burning wine."

Delicious, yes. But can it help relieve cramps, too? You bet, according to experts. Prepared mustard contains vinegar and sodium, the same muscle-soothing ingredients found in sports drinks and the trendy cramp-reliever, pickle juice. And bright yellow turmeric — added to give mustard its appealing color — is bursting with anti-inflammatory properties that might be just what the doctor ordered for your late-night muscle cramps.

A couple of teaspoons is all you need to stop a charley horse in its tracks.

Manage muscle pain with heat. Use a hot compress or heating pad to help relax your tight muscles.

Make a simple compress by dampening a towel with warm water. Apply to the affected area for 15 to 20 minutes, three or four times a day.

If using a heating pad, be sure to protect yourself from burns. Never place it directly on your skin. And be especially careful if you have nerve damage from diabetes or other medical conditions.

Rx Alert

One toxic tonic?

Quinine was the go-to treatment for leg-cramp sufferers for decades. Then in 2006, reports of serious side effects — including a deadly blood disorder — forced the FDA to ban all drug products containing quinine, save one, Qualaquin, which is only approved to treat malaria.

You can still get a small amount of quinine in tonic water, though — it's the ingredient that adds that bitter taste. And while drinking a few ounces shouldn't be harmful, it's also not likely to prevent your leg cramps.

Nausea

A throbbing headache. A stomach bug. New medications. Just about anything can bring on a bad case of the queasies. And once your stomach starts to roll, you'll do whatever it takes to make it stop.

This need to purge is not a disease by itself, but rather a symptom of something else going on in your body. Figuring that out will help you, and your doctor, determine the correct treatment.

Why, oh why do you feel so sick? Often nausea is simply part of another condition, like a migraine or a food allergy. Other times, it's a sign of something more serious like cancer, an intestinal blockage, or glaucoma.

It's also a common side effect of certain changes in your body — pregnancy, low blood sugar, or anesthesia from a surgical procedure. Even bingeing on fatty foods or chugging too much caffeine or alcohol can make you feel like losing your lunch.

Take the edge off your tummy troubles. Not sure why you're nauseous? Then you may want to visit your doctor, especially if you're in severe pain or if you've been vomiting for over 24 hours and can't hold down any liquids.

On the other hand, if you suffer from an occasional bout and you're sure it's nothing serious, try simple home remedies like these to get you through:

▶ Sip plenty of water.

▶ Avoid coffee and caffeinated colas.

▸ Eat bland foods.

▸ Steer clear of spicy and fried fare.

▸ Stay away from strong smells like perfumes, cigarette smoke, and pungent foods.

Then add the following to your anti-nausea arsenal.

3 natural ways to quit feeling queasy

Rub on relief with soothing herbs. When your body tells you it's going to be sick, tell your body you'd rather try an herbal massage, instead.

▸ **Fennel.** Herbalists swear by this fragrant remedy, saying it offers fast relief. Mix a few drops of fennel essential oil with a tablespoon of olive oil in a bowl. Rub on your belly, then cover for several minutes with a moist heating pad set on low or medium. Repeat every two to three hours.

▸ **Coriander.** Mix eight drops of coriander essential oil with a tablespoon of olive oil. Test on a small patch of skin and, if you don't react, massage into your arms, legs, back, chest, and tummy. This seems especially effective for nausea associated with a migraine headache. Repeat as needed.

Hydrate to shrink healing time. Truthfully, almost any liquid will help, since experts say staying hydrated is key to feeling better faster. But a soothing cup of herbal tea will do wonders to settle your stomach and prevent nausea and vomiting.

Chamomile relaxes your muscles and relieves stomach flu symptoms, while ginger, an herb given as a token of love centuries ago, gives back a little love to your upset tummy two ways. It calms the stomach flu by fighting off the virus that causes it, while quelling nausea and vomiting. You'll find chamomile and ginger teas at most supermarkets.

You can also stay hydrated with any of the following:

▸ carbonated drinks, decaffeinated and nonalcoholic

▸ two teaspoons fresh lemon juice mixed in a glass of water

▸ apple juice

▸ ice pops

▸ clear broth or bouillon

▸ sports drinks

▸ gelatin

▸ ice chips

▸ flat ginger ale

▸ coconut water

> You can't see them, but microscopic bugs could be living on your strawberries, spinach, pears, or other produce, just waiting to make you sick. Don't worry — it takes two quick steps to get your fruits and vegetables virtually free of *E. coli*, *Salmonella*, and other food bugs. Spray with a mild vinegar solution, then rinse for 30 seconds.

Get a whiff of these "scent"sational remedies. It's the difference between a garbage dump and a dozen roses. Some smells make you sick to your stomach while others refresh you. Inhale any of the following fragrances and you may find a natural cure to that icky sensation in the pit of your stomach.

▸ **Grapefruit.** Make your own smelling salts by mixing two tablespoons sea salt with 10 to 12 drops of grapefruit essential oil in a dark-colored bottle. Shake well to blend. Inhale as needed to settle any queasiness you're experiencing.

▸ **Anise.** The seeds from this flowering plant have a sharp aroma similar to licorice and have been used since ancient times in medicine, cosmetics, and cooking. To ease your nausea, place one or two drops of the essential oil on a tissue and hold in front of your nose. Or take a whiff directly from the bottle. Just don't come in contact with the oil if you have sensitive skin. It can cause a rash.

▸ **Spearmint, peppermint, ginger, and cardamom blend.** Mix several essential oils for an aromatherapy bouquet that will soothe your sick stomach. People suffering from post-operative nausea who inhaled this combination felt less sick, found one study.

▸ **Lemon.** When life gives you lemons, take a whiff! Lemon essential oil lessened nausea and vomiting in pregnant women, according to Iranian researchers. Give this simple remedy a try to see if it helps you feel better, too.

▸ **Isopropyl alcohol.** Emergency room patients in Texas experiencing nausea received pads saturated with either isopropyl alcohol or a simple saline solution. Those who sniffed the alcohol pads were twice as likely to feel relief compared to the saline sniffers. Participants inhaled a total of three times, two minutes apart.

"Nausea and vomiting are the chief complaint for nearly 5 million emergency patients every year," said lead study author Kenneth Beadle, of the San Antonio Uniformed Services Health Education Consortium in San Antonio. He believes this cheap, easy, and fast remedy has the potential to help a lot of people.

Osteoarthritis

Got a bum knee? Stiff shoulder? Swollen fingers? You're not alone. Over 50 million Americans have some type of arthritis, the leading cause of disability in the U.S. It can make taking the stairs, lifting that grandbaby, or opening a jar of pickles awkward on your best days, downright impossible on others.

But what exactly is this disease that causes your bony hinges to howl? Simply put, arthritis refers to many kinds of joint pain or joint disease. In fact, there are over 100 types and related conditions, but osteoarthritis (OA) is the most common.

With OA, your cartilage, the flexible cushion between your bones, breaks apart, and bone starts to rub against bone. The result — pain, swelling, and stiffness. Your joints may become deformed and you can find it hard to move and perform daily tasks.

Experts say it's unclear why people get OA, but it's often the result of aging, being overweight, a previous injury, or simple genetics. There's also no cure for it, so your first course of action is to prevent it.

The weather really can trigger arthritis agony. People with OA felt more discomfort when the temperature was low or the humidity was high, shows one study. Researchers think it's because a drop in air pressure causes tissues to swell, increasing pain. Or perhaps when it's cold and rainy, you simply don't spend enough time exercising to loosen your joints up.

- Maintain a healthy weight.

- Get off the couch and start exercising.

- Mix up movements, especially when you work out, to avoid too much repetition on a single joint.

- Avoid situations that may lead to joint injuries.

Once OA sets in, all is not lost. There's plenty you can do to turn down the dial on your pain meter.

8 ways to knock out arthritis pain

Feast on a fabulous fat. Take note. Not all fats are bad for you.

Omega-3 fatty acids, for instance, are considered essential fatty acids because, although your body needs them — to form healthy cells, promote a healthy brain and nervous system, and support your immune function — you cannot make them. You must get omega 3 from food.

Not to mention, omega-3 fatty acids fight inflammation by blocking two of your body's chemicals — cytokines and prostaglandins — that trigger inflammation. And that makes it an OA superstar.

Its cousin, omega-6, is also essential, but this fatty acid affects your health in a different way. Too much omega-6 raises inflammation.

Your best bet is to balance the two fats. Experts suggest that for every 4 grams of omega-6 in your diet, you should try to eat 1 gram of omega-3. Unfortunately, most folks in developed countries like the United States miss that mark by a long shot, getting as many as 30 grams of omega-6 for every one of omega-3. That's because people eat too much meat and processed foods, which tend to be high in omega-6, and too little fish, flaxseed, and canola oil, which are rich in omega-3.

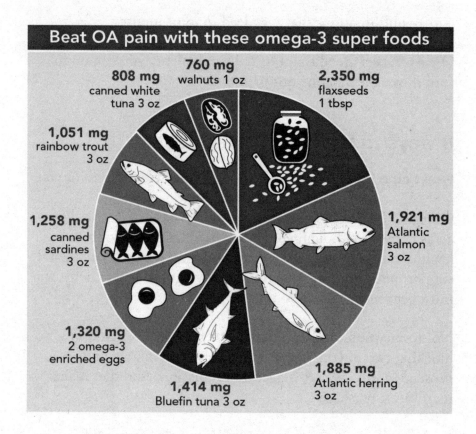

It's time to switch things up if you want to ease your achy joints. While you can get omega-3 in a fish oil supplement, scientists say getting it from food is better. Try the nine super sources shown above that are proven to get rid of joint pain and increase mobility.

Water aerobics: OA fitness in the fast lane. Find something that makes you want to move, and just do it. That's what experts say is the key to soothing sore joints. And the more you move, the less likely you are to suffer serious joint limitations as you age.

But what if you can't imagine working out because you're in too much pain? Consider diving into a water aerobics class or one featuring resistance exercises in the pool. Not only will you place less stress on your joints, but you could actually improve the health of your cartilage.

Finnish researchers discovered this when women with knee arthritis took part in four months of high-intensity resistance training in the water — one hour, three times a week. And they meant high-intensity. The workouts were vigorous enough to really get their hearts pumping, with 400 to 500 repetitions per session.

Sip green tea for sweet relief. Not only will a warm cup of green tea soothe your soul, it will give your achy joints peace and comfort, too.

And that's because green tea is swimming in polyphenols — natural plant chemicals praised by doctors as useful for preventing and treating osteoarthritis.

Epigallocatechin gallate (EGCG), for example, is one polyphenol in green tea that controls inflammation. Others block the production of a compound in your body, nitric oxide. And that, essentially, stops your cartilage from breaking down. Polyphenols also protect your collagen, the connective tissue found in bones, tendons, and ligaments.

Not bad for a humble cup of tea.

Soothe foot aches with "sole" mates. Goodbye foot pain. Hello orthotics, therapeutic shoe inserts proven to relieve arthritis.

Whether you have OA pain in a toe joint, your ankle, knee, or hip, orthotics can help, say experts at the Arthritis Foundation. These cushioned inserts relieve pressure by buffering sensitive areas and distributing your weight differently. They can even change the way you walk.

Australian researchers confirmed this when they tested people with arthritis in their big toe. The orthotics helped by shifting pressure away from the painful joint and toward the arch and other toes.

If you're looking for shoe inserts to minimize your pain, experts offer these helpful tips.

▸ Insoles should feel comfortable as soon as you start using them. Check them out on both feet before buying.

▸ Trim them to fit, if necessary. No buckling or wrinkling allowed.

▸ Take your insoles with you when shopping for new shoes.

▸ There's no need to pay big bucks for custom-made insoles. You can pick up a pair of ready-to-wear orthotics at your local drugstore without a prescription.

Give heat a warm welcome. Nothing makes you go "ahhh" like the feeling of warmth on your stiff joints. Say hello to these toasty tips, so you can say bye-bye to aches and pains.

▸ Don't wait until winter to take advantage of an electric blanket. Use it year-round and set it to come on shortly before it's time to get up in the morning. The heat will loosen you up before you climb out of bed.

▸ When OA pain cripples your fingers, head to the kitchen. Run six to eight inches of hot water in your sink, slide on dishwashing gloves, and immerse your hands in the water for five or 10 minutes. You'll feel like you are spoiling yourself at a spa. For extra comfort, rub mineral oil on your hands before putting on the gloves.

▸ Make your own moist heating pad by placing a wet towel in a freezer bag and microwaving it. Carefully remove from the microwave — watch out, it's hot! — by wrapping another towel around it. Lay over sore spots for 15 to 20 minutes.

Brace yourself for pain-free knees. A little support can go a long way when it comes to your knees. Simply strapping on a brace can work miracles. Generally speaking there are two types.

▸ One is a sleeve you pull up over your knee, available at local drugstores and sporting goods centers. Sleeve braces provide stability while still allowing good movement. People who wore a flexible Lycra knee brace for about seven hours a day felt less pain after six weeks than those who didn't wear one, found a study out of the United Kingdom. What's more, wearing a brace also healed some of the tiny fractures below the bone surface typically found in arthritic knees. For under $20, you can give this over-the-counter brace a try and see if it offers the support you need.

▸ Another type of brace is custom-made, with plastic and steel supports. Called an unloader brace, it takes the pressure off your knee joint and places it on the thigh bone. This forces your knee to bend away from the painful area. Unloader braces support knees with advanced arthritis and may help delay replacement surgery. They require a prescription and can be costly if your insurance doesn't cover them.

Build better joints and battle arthritis with broccoli. Why settle for the same old side dish when you can have broccoli, a vegetable superfood that protects the cartilage in your joints.

Broccoli contains sulforaphane, a natural chemical that, according to a study out of the University of Oxford in England, blocks inflammation by shutting down joint-damaging enzymes.

While sulforaphane is also found in a number of other cruciferous vegetables, like Brussels sprouts and cabbage, if you want a tasty and healthy way to ease stiffness and OA pain, just say, "Pass the broccoli!"

Nosh on these "berry" natural pain killers. Eat a bowl of berries today, and you'll fight inflammation for a day. Eat a bowl every day, and you'll guard against arthritis for a lifetime.

That's because berries are low in calories and high in antioxidants and phytochemicals, natural compounds that fight disease and inflammation. They also lower C-reactive protein, a measure of inflammation in your blood and a compound linked to arthritis.

Specifically, berries are chock-full of anthocyanins, the phytochemicals that give strawberries, blueberries, raspberries, and açai berries their rich colors and anti-inflammatory powers. In addition, cranberries contain proanthocyanidins, another type of natural anti-inflammatory.

Flaxseed crusted fish

Recipe

Ease your pain with this easy weeknight dinner
that can repair damaged joints — featuring five fabulous
Bible foods.

Take your favorite fatty fish, maybe mackerel or salmon,
drizzle with extra virgin olive oil, then sprinkle generously
with garlic and ground flaxseed or flaxseed meal. Bake
or broil until the fish is flaky, and serve topped with
toasted walnuts.

If you prefer you can dredge your fish in a little milk or
beaten egg first, then coat with a mixture of bread crumbs,
finely chopped nuts, and flaxseeds. Pan fry it with garlic
and olive oil.

Make this a weekly favorite, and you'll get plenty of omega-
3 fatty acids from the fish, flaxseeds, and walnuts; antioxidants from the garlic; and oleocanthal from the olive oil —
a meal full of all-natural anti-inflammatories.

Beat arthritis with these must-have nutrients

Want a lifetime of happy joints? Look no further than these
seven super nutrients.

Calcium. Ninety-nine percent of your body's calcium is in
your skeleton, proving just how vital this mineral is to strong
bones. Make sure you get the 1,000 to 1,200 milligrams (mg)
you need daily from dairy products and foods fortified with
calcium. For better absorption, get plenty of vitamin D and
phosphorus, too.

Magnesium. This magnificent mineral promotes tendon and cartilage function, and works hand-in-hand with calcium to boost bone mineral density. Eat nuts, beans, and whole grains to get the recommended daily requirements — 320 mg for women and 420 mg for men.

Phosphorus. With 85 percent of all phosphorus found in your skeleton, it's no surprise this mineral is necessary for joint health. Eat phosphorus-rich foods like milk, cheese, seeds, nuts, fortified cereals, meat, fish, and poultry to get the recommended 700 mg a day.

Protein. You probably think of protein as something your muscles need. And you would be right. But your joints need it, too, since protein gives shape and strength to your bones and tendons. Experts recommend about 7 grams (g) of protein for every 20 pounds of body weight, or approximately 46 g for women and 56 g for men every day.

Vitamin C. The C could stand for "critical" because this vitamin plays a crucial role in bone and cartilage growth. Studies show vitamin C lowers the risk of cartilage loss and can keep your OA from getting worse. Fruits and vegetables like kiwi, oranges, grapefruit, red and green bell peppers, and cantaloupes are just a few of the best sources. Men should get 90 mg daily and women 75 mg.

Vitamin D. The jury seems out on this one. While vitamin D is definitely important for bone strength, it may not directly improve your OA symptoms — unless your D levels are low to start with. Adults should get from 600 to 800 international units (IU) daily. Although your body can make vitamin D from sunshine, you can only get it from fortified milk and a few other foods, like fish. Talk to your doctor about taking supplements.

Zinc. You may not hear as much about zinc as you do calcium and magnesium, but when it comes to joint health, this trace mineral is essential. Studies show people with osteoarthritis have low levels of zinc. Men need 11 mg daily and women need 8 mg. Get zinc from milk, cheese, pork, red meat, whole-grain cereals, and dark chicken meat.

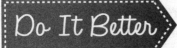

Do It Better   Make your life easier every day

When joint pain gets you down, try these quick and easy ways to get things done around the house.

- Use a lightweight leaf blower instead of a shovel to blast away powdery snow.

- Slip on microfiber gloves to dust shelves and furniture.

- Get rid of knickknacks around the house. The less you have to clean, the better.

- Turn on your cellphone speaker, then put your phone down when you make or take calls.

- Toss your dirty clothes into a rolling laundry cart instead of a basket.

- Wear neckties that come pre-tied.

- Use "power" tools like a battery-operated tooth-brush, or a kitchen mixer instead of a whisk.

Work out to work through joint pain

"The one thing that can solve most of our problems," said iconic funk and soul musician James Brown, "is dancing." You better believe this Godfather of Soul knew what he was talking about, because dancing is, indeed, one sure way to solve a host of health issues. Swing it, tango to it, or just shimmy and shake, and you'll not only give your muscles and your heart a workout, but you'll boost your brain and your mood, as well. What about those achy joints?

Go ahead. Get your dancing shoes on. You'll ease OA pain while strengthening the muscles that support your joints. Shoot for 45 minutes of dancing twice a week and you may find yourself walking faster while feeling less hip and knee discomfort. Consider taking a low-impact class, like ballroom dancing, Jazzercise Lite, or Zumba for older adults.

So what activity makes you feel better? Because whatever that is, you need to start doing it every day to battle arthritis woes. "The more you do each day, the better your knees will support you," says Dr. Suzanne Salamon in the Harvard University publication *Staying Healthy and Independent for Life*.

So why not add something active to your daily routine? Any of the following will keep you footloose and fancy-free.

Balance training. To increase mobility, especially if you've had knee surgery, try balance exercises. Stand on one leg for 10 seconds, then switch sides. Work up to one minute on each leg. Do these near a counter in case you need to catch yourself. Also, practice standing up from a chair without using your hands.

Hand exercises. Strengthen your grip, increase hand mobility, and reduce finger and wrist pain with your own at-home therapy. Three times a week, take a rubber ball, spread your fingers wide around it, then roll them into a fist. Start with 10 repetitions and work up to 15.

Warning

OA: the hidden heart threat

There's a relationship between arthritis and heart disease — and it's not a good one.

Multiple studies show people with OA are at higher risk for heart attack and are more likely to be hospitalized for heart-related issues.

Although experts aren't sure why there's a connection, some suspect inflammation is part of the picture. More importantly though, people suffering from OA increase their risk of heart disease because they:

- are more likely to be overweight.

- are less likely to exercise.

- often take nonsteroidal anti-inflammatory drugs (NSAIDs) for pain.

The good news is these are all things you can change. And while it's too early to tell if people with OA need to be checked above and beyond regular heart disease screenings, for now, continue to exercise. This will strengthen your heart, lower high blood pressure and cholesterol, and slash soreness.

Jumping. Sounds counterintuitive, but Finnish scientists discovered improvement in knee cartilage and mobility in postmenopausal women with mild arthritis in their knees who performed high-impact jumping exercises three times a week. Surprisingly, 12 months of jump training did not trigger pain or stiffness.

Strength and range-of-motion training. Don't let arthritis in your hips stop you from working out. Both water and land-based exercises helped people with hip OA manage their pain, found a review of several studies. Moving, bending, and stretching a joint in different directions will keep it flexible, while working against weights or stretch bands will gently strengthen the muscles that support your joints. Experts say a 12-week program, working out three times a week should help.

Tai chi. The beautiful, flowing movements of this ancient martial art not only relieve stress and anxiety, they ease the pain and stiffness of osteoarthritis. Researchers looked at data from 33 studies and found that tai chi generally improved quality of life for people with OA, making it easier for them to get up and go.

And the *Annals of Internal Medicine* reports people with knee arthritis who did tai chi twice a week for 12 weeks had less pain and improved mobility — as much as people who underwent traditional physical therapy.

Walking. Experts agree walking is good for people with arthritis. You maintain your weight while improving your balance and heart health. Plus, walking builds bone strength and maintains bone density. Start by walking 10 minutes a day and work up to 35 to 40 minutes a day.

Yoga. People all over the U.S. practice yoga every day, and it's especially helpful if you have OA in your knees, say experts. "Yoga may be especially well suited to people with arthritis because it combines physical activity with potent stress management and relaxation techniques, and focuses on respecting limitations that can change from day to day," says Dr. Susan J. Bartlett, associate professor at Johns Hopkins School of Medicine in Baltimore.

Rx Alert

Trade your pain meds for these savory spices

Nonsteroidal anti-inflammatory drugs, known as NSAIDs, have long been the go-to remedy for OA pain. But maybe they shouldn't be. Taking these drugs, available with or without a prescription, can raise your ulcer risk as well as your blood pressure. What's more, COX-2 inhibitors, the newest NSAIDs for arthritis, bump up the threat of heart attack.

When it comes to OA pain, why take something that can hurt you when you can take something that can help — even heal you?

Ginger. Adding one-fourth to one-half teaspoon of ginger to your daily diet can slash the pain and disability associated with OA, say experts. Plus, ginger heals your stomach lining, unlike NSAIDs that can damage it.

Turmeric. It's the tasty spice that gives curry and mustard their golden color. But what makes turmeric a powerful pain reliever? A phytonutrient, called curcumin. Thai scientists tested this natural plant chemical against ibuprofen in people with knee OA. After six weeks, the curcumin group felt as much pain relief as the pill poppers.

Osteoporosis

Remember the dusty skeleton hanging in your high school biology class oh-so-many years ago? That guy will look just the same if you pay him a visit during your next reunion. *Your* bones, on the other hand, have changed quite a bit.

Back in your school days, they were close to being the strongest and most dense they would ever be. Since then, they've gone through decades of remodeling, a process where bone cells dissolve and new ones form. In fact, about 10 percent of your skeleton is replaced through remodeling every year.

At least, that's how it's supposed to work. But sometimes, because of hormone levels, nutrient deficiencies, medications, or lifestyle, more cells break down than are created. When that happens, your bones develop a network of tiny holes, like Swiss cheese. This is known as low bone density, or osteopenia. If it worsens, it can eventually develop into osteoporosis, where your bones become even more fragile and likely to fracture.

The National Institutes of Health estimates that 10 million Americans have osteoporosis, with another 43 million at high risk. Who, exactly, is this disease most likely to hit? Older, white women who are slender and have a family history of osteoporosis. But regardless of your age or gender — take note, over 2 million men have osteoporosis — talk to your doctor about screening for this bone disease if you:

▶ begin to lose height.

▸ suffer from back pain.

▸ develop a stooped posture.

He may order a bone mineral density (BMD) test or a bone measurement, also known as dual X-ray absorptiometry (DXA) scan.

Since you may never know you suffer from brittle bones until one breaks, it's especially important to diagnosis this "silent disease" early. With osteoporosis, your chances of hip, spine, and wrist fractures go up. And new research shows that half of older folks who fracture a hip will never be as active and independent as they were before.

Luckily, you can strengthen your body naturally and cut down your risk of breakable bones.

8 super strategies to build strong bones

Fill up on bone-building nutrients. You need calcium in your bloodstream to carry out important jobs, like transmit nerve impulses, contract muscles, and control when your blood vessels narrow and relax. But 99 percent of the calcium in your body is in your bones and teeth. So when you don't have enough extra calcium to perform all these tasks, you "borrow" it from your bones. You can see how that is a problem.

So the more calcium, the better, right? Not necessarily. Researchers out of New Zealand looked at nearly 30 years' worth of studies involving men and women over age 50, how much calcium they got from either food or supplements, and their risk of fractures. The bottom line — while experts say you need 1,200 milligrams of calcium each day, they did not find getting more will protect your bones.

And talk to your doctor before you turn to calcium supplements anyway, because they come with risks, including heart attack, stroke, dementia, digestive problems, and kidney stones.

No bones about it, the best way to get this important mineral is through your diet. But remember, there's more to bone health than just calcium. Here are some of the nutrients you should be getting every day — and why.

Nutrient	Food Sources	Action
Calcium	yogurt, collard greens, milk, broccoli	builds and maintains bones
Magnesium	bran cereal, brown rice, almonds, mackerel	may increase bone mineral density
Omega-3 fatty acids	salmon, walnuts, herring, sardines, flaxseeds	makes calcium more available
Potassium	baked potato, prunes, raisins, lima beans, bananas	prevents bone breakdown
Vitamin C	oranges, broccoli, strawberries, sweet red peppers	helps make collagen, which forms the framework of bone
Vitamin D	salmon, tuna, fortified cereals	helps your body absorb calcium
Vitamin K1	Swiss chard, kale, broccoli, spinach	binds calcium to bones
Vitamin K2	cheese, egg yolks, fermented soybeans, chicken liver	helps build stronger bones

Feast on fruits and vegetables packed with antioxidants.
You've heard of them. Those powerful little nutrients that landed

blueberries in the superfood category. But do you really know what they do?

When your body processes the oxygen you breathe, it also produces free radicals, unstable molecules that lack one electron. Because they are unbalanced, these free radicals travel through your body, like a band of pickpockets, trying to steal electrons from stable, healthy cells. When they succeed, they leave the cell irreversibly damaged.

One damaged cell is no big deal. But over time, lots of these pickpocket molecules can cause so much damage, called oxidation, that your body becomes weak. In fact, researchers have linked free radical damage to over 200 diseases — including osteoporosis.

Luckily, you can stop the damage with antioxidants. They fight oxidation by combining with free radicals or giving them an electron, to make them stable. Your body produces some antioxidants itself, but you can also get loads of them from fresh fruits and vegetables.

Turns out, two unassuming foods have high antioxidant power and are proven to slow bone loss.

The first unlikely hero is the dried plum. Commonly known as a prune, it might just be the next superfood of the fruit world. It's cheap. It's sweet. And researchers are surprised at just how much disease-fighting power it has.

Its success is due to polyphenols, natural plant chemicals known for their antioxidant and anti-inflammatory powers. These guys boost bone formation and block bone loss. One recent study showed benefits from just a single serving a day
— that's about five prunes.

And don't forget about the ordinary — but extraordinary — tomato. It contains lycopene, another natural compound that fights oxidation. When researchers gave postmenopausal women lycopene for four months, either in tomato juice or supplements, they found it reduced bone breakdown and increased bone strength. The study used at least 30 milligrams (mg) of lycopene a day, roughly the amount you'll find in a cup of spaghetti sauce or tomato juice. You can also get lycopene in other red fruits and vegetables like guavas, watermelon, and sweet red peppers.

Warning

Bad-to-the-bone beverages block calcium

Spinach, rhubarb, and beet greens may be healthy, calcium-rich vegetables, but they come with a little hitch. Oxalates. This natural compound keeps your body from fully absorbing the calcium.

Watch out for other items, like some of your favorite drinks, containing ingredients that also block this important nutrient.

- **Energy drinks.** Sodium in these deplete calcium and cause bone loss.

- **Coffee and tea.** These breakfast favorites naturally contain caffeine, which seems to lower how much calcium your body absorbs.

- **Soft drinks.** Many colas contain caffeine and phosphorus, which have been linked to bone loss.

- **Alcohol.** It may also lower your calcium levels. Plus drinking is related to falls and broken bones.

Buck up your bones with resistance training. When astronauts go into space they face a serious problem. In the weightless environment, their bodies don't get enough action, and they begin to lose bone and muscle. So what do they do?

Well, according to NASA, they spend two-and-a-half hours every day exercising, in an attempt to fight this decline. One of their three pieces of equipment is a Resistance Exercise Device, because weight-bearing physical activity causes new bone tissue to form. Folks who lift weights simply have stronger bones.

Here on Earth, it's much easier to score the benefits of resistance training. And you don't have to be a heavyweight champion, either. Research published in *The Journal of Sports Medicine and Physical Fitness* says you can still increase bone density using light weights if you go for a longer workout.

Even better news, those in the study already suffering from osteopenia saw this type of exercise program increase their bone mineral density by 29 percent. Grab a couple of cans from your pantry and start pumping iron.

It takes guts to build healthy bones. Soluble corn fiber. You've probably never heard of it, but you're certainly eating it. SCF is a corn product that's been used in a variety of processed foods since 2007, to sweeten without added sugar, and to pump up fiber content. You might see it listed as maltodextrin in cereals, baked goods, candy, dairy products, frozen foods, soups, salad dressings, fruit drinks, carbonated beverages, meal replacement drinks, and flavored water.

So why do you and your bones care about SCF? Because it's a prebiotic that affects the pH in your large intestines, prompting your body to absorb more calcium and increase bone density. In fact, a study recently published in the *American Journal of Clinical Nutrition* said 20 grams of soluble corn fiber a day for 50 days actually boosted calcium absorption by 7 percent.

"If projected out for a year, this would equal and counter the average rate of bone loss in a postmenopausal woman," said Connie Weaver, distinguished professor at Purdue University and part of the research team.

"Most studies looking at benefits from soluble corn fiber are trying to solve digestion problems, and we are the first to determine that this relationship of feeding certain kinds of fiber can alter the gut microbiome in ways that can enhance health," Weaver said. "We found this prebiotic can help healthy people use minerals better to support bone health."

You can buy soluble corn fiber as a supplement, but talk to your doctor before making it part of your daily routine.

Spice up bone health with turmeric. It may be the golden spice of India, but this colorful seasoning is trending all over the U.S. And its health benefits aren't all hype. The turmeric plant has a special ingredient called curcumin that could battle bone loss.

Dozens of studies show curcumin supports your skeleton in a number of ways. It may:

▶ bump up antioxidant activity to defend your body against free radical damage.

▶ activate vitamin D receptors, which help keep calcium in your bones.

▶ prevent the breakdown of bone and encourage the formation of new bone.

Some experiments even show that curcumin can fight bone loss related to menopause and steroid therapy.

Because these studies have been on mice, researchers aren't ready to recommend a dose for people. But add turmeric to rice, condiments, sautéed vegetables, and more to make your taste buds and your bones happy.

Snack on soybeans to reinforce bone strength. As if hot flashes, dry hair, and insomnia aren't enough, menopause can trigger another symptom — bone loss.

During this change of life, women produce less estrogen, a hormone that protects bones. Without it, osteoporosis is a much bigger threat. Amazingly, some foods contain natural chemicals called isoflavones that are similar in structure to these hormones and may mimic their estrogen-like effects. You can get a small amount from certain grains and vegetables, but soybeans are by far the best source.

The research on soy isoflavones and bone health — particularly in menopausal women — is a mixed bag. Many studies show stronger bones and less bone loss, while others do not. Some experts say whether or not soy works for you could depend on how your body processes it. And that could depend on things like the amount and type of bacteria in your intestines. Only about a third of the people in Western countries seem to process soy into a component that helps their bones.

If you're going to try soy, get no more than three to five servings a day and eat whole foods that are less processed, like edamame, tofu, tempeh, miso, and natto. If it says "soy protein" on the label, loads of nutrients have been removed.

Some research links soy to an increased risk of health problems such as stroke and dementia, so ask your doctor if it's a good choice for you.

Prevent bone loss with a little help from gravity. You've heard of Newton's laws and maybe even Murphy's law, but Wolff's law probably isn't on your radar. Maybe it should be.

This law states when you change how you use a bone, its physical structure changes, too. Put more stress or weight on it, and, over time, your bone becomes denser and stronger. And that's why some types of exercise improve bone health better than others. They are called weight-bearing or load-bearing activities, and they use your body weight to make you work against gravity.

They can be high-impact workouts, like dancing, running, and jumping rope; low-impact, like speed walking and using an elliptical machine; or a sport, like tennis, soccer, and basketball. Even a few minutes of hopping a day can mean stronger bones that are more resistant to fractures.

The force put on your skeleton by these weight-bearing exercises encourages new bone tissue to grow, strengthening your frame and possibly preventing osteoporosis. Just ask your doctor about your fracture risk and if weight-bearing exercises are safe for you.

Say no to drugs by saying yes to beans. It's old advice — beans are a no-no when it comes to your bones. Animal studies from decades ago claimed phytates, natural compounds in beans, whole grains, and nuts, were bad for bones because they interfered with how you absorb minerals like calcium. But more recent studies on people say this just isn't so.

In fact, the research shows bone mineral density increases when you eat more phytates. This could be because phytates limit the number of cells that break down your bones. Scientists out of Spain measured bone density in the spine, hip, and heel of more than 1,800 volunteers, and found the more phytates in their diet, the stronger their bones. It seems that not getting enough phytates is actually an osteoporosis risk factor.

Michael Greger, M.D., author of *How Not to Die,* points out there are reports saying phytates can slow the breakdown of bone, very much like the anti-osteoporosis drug Fosamax — but without the risk of side effects.

Is breakfast wrecking your bones?

If cereal is your go-to breakfast, you may be damaging your bones without even realizing it. That's because you're getting a heaping helping of the mineral phosphorus.

Why do you care? Because too much phosphorus causes your body to pull calcium out of your bones, making them weak.

Keep tabs on phosphorus to maintain brawny bones. Make no mistake, your body needs phosphorus. In fact, it's necessary for your cells and tissues to grow and repair themselves.

But getting enough is not a problem. It occurs naturally in most animal and plant foods, including dairy products, meat, fish, legumes, nuts, seeds, and even chocolate. Your body will absorb, at most, 60 percent of the organic phosphorus in these foods. But wait. There's more.

Phosphorus, in the form of phosphates, is also an ingredient in many food additives, used to boost flavor, increase moisture, and change the color of foods. A study published in the *Journal of Renal Nutrition* found there were phosphorus-containing food additives in 44 percent of the best-selling grocery items. And the worst news is you absorb more of this type of inorganic phosphate — up to 100 percent.

The recommended dietary allowance (RDA) of phosphorus is 700 milligrams (mg) a day. Yet, because so much phosphorus is hidden in processed foods, experts say men get an average of 1,602 mg daily, and women 1,128 mg. If you eat a lot of processed foods, you could even approach the maximum safe amount of 4,000 mg a day.

Channel your inner Sherlock to spot sneaky additives. The FDA doesn't require manufacturers to list phosphorus levels on packaging. So for now, one of the best ways to spot added phosphorus is to look for the letters "phos" in the ingredient list. Popular additives include dicalcium phosphate, monosodium phosphate, and phosphoric acid.

Besides milk and cereal, these processed foods contain added phosphorus.

- bread and baked goods

- canned iced tea

- cheese

- cocoa and other chocolate drinks

- dark colas and many other bottled beverages

▸ dry food mixes

▸ ice cream

▸ liquid nondairy creamer

▸ prepared frozen foods

▸ processed meats

▸ pudding

Stem cell therapy reverses bone damage

New!

Imagine a single injection that could restore your aging bones. That's what stem cell researchers are proposing in their latest investigation.

The recent study showed that a shot of stem cells from healthy mice transformed unhealthy bone in mice with osteoporosis.

"We had hoped for a general increase in bone health," said John E. Davies, Professor at the University of Toronto and a co-author of the study. "But the huge surprise was to find that the exquisite inner 'coral-like' architecture of the bone structure of the injected animals — which is severely compromised in osteoporosis — was restored to normal."

Researchers hope they will be able to use this new technology in the future to prevent age-related osteoporosis in people.

Sinusitis

Americans spend over $6 billion every year on sinusitis treatments. That's almost enough to give every man, woman, and child in the country a crisp $20 bill. Sadly, most of that money is wasted. Antibiotics are rarely needed for sinusitis, and many over-the-counter drugs just make your symptoms worse in the long run. The best relief comes from simple, at-home treatments.

Sinusitis is really just inflammation of your sinuses and nasal passages. The membrane lining your sinuses produces mucus, which normally flows out through your nose. When something irritates that membrane, like a cold virus, allergies, cigarette smoke, or bacteria, it swells. The swelling blocks the exit route to your nose, trapping air and mucus in your sinuses. As the mucus gets thicker, bacteria may start to flourish, setting the stage for a secondary infection.

> Up to 98 percent of sinusitis cases are caused by viruses. That means antibiotics rarely help you get better. But if you have a fever over 102 degrees, your symptoms suddenly get worse, or you don't feel better after 10 days, you need to go to your doctor for antibiotics.

Learn to spot sinusitis. Your stuffy nose, sneezing, coughing, sore throat, and facial pressure could be caused by a sinus infection. Or you could have a cold, the flu, or allergies. So how can you tell the difference?

You should suspect you have sinusitis if your symptoms get worse over time and last longer than a week. Sinusitis may give you a headache first thing in the morning, painful sinus pressure at night, or head pain when you bend over. Your nasal discharge might be yellowish-green or gray, and you may have a sore throat from postnasal drip.

How long will the misery last? There are four different types of sinusitis, each classified by how long the infection persists.

▶ Acute lasts less than four weeks.

▶ Subacute lasts between four and 12 weeks.

▶ Chronic sinusitis lasts three months or longer.

▶ If you have more than three episodes in one year, you have recurrent sinusitis.

If you've ever dealt with a nasty sinus infection, you know even a couple of weeks is too long to wait for relief. Follow these simple tips to stop sinus problems in their tracks.

5 ways to say so long to sinus suffering

Fight fire with fire — use bacteria to stop sinus troubles.
Bacteria have gotten a bad rap. You probably just think of them as germs. And, in some cases, you would be right. But the bacteria that live and thrive inside your body are so much more. They affect everything from your allergies to your blood pressure. So researchers have turned to probiotics, which are microorganisms similar to the ones you have naturally in your body, as a way to stop sinus problems without a single drug.

Your sinuses are home to millions of microorganisms, both good and bad. Swiss researchers found that drinking probiotic fermented milk daily for three weeks lowered the number of disease-causing bacteria in the nose. This helps fight off sinusitis, as well as other infections like colds and pneumonia.

If you can't find probiotic fermented milk at the grocery store, don't worry. Look for yogurt, like Activia, or granola bars, cereals, and juices that contain probiotics.

In order to get all the benefits from probiotics, check the label for the number of colony forming units, or CFUs, a product has. Aim for at least 5 to 10 billion per serving.

While you can always try supplements, ask your doctor first.

Spicy tomato tonic

Some experts think a spiced drink like this one may help clear up sinus congestion.

> 8 oz low-sodium tomato juice
> 1 tsp chopped garlic
> 3/4 tsp lemon juice
> 1/4 tsp Tabasco sauce

Mix together, heat until warm, and sip slowly.

Clear your nose with these superfoods. What do apples, blackberries, onions, blueberries, broccoli, and kale have in common? They're all packed with a naturally occurring chemical called quercetin that fights inflammation.

Not only can it help soothe your inflamed sinuses, quercetin blocks the release of histamines that can cause allergy symptoms and irritate your nose.

If you're having trouble getting enough quercetin through your diet, ask your doctor if supplements are right for you.

Rinse away stuffiness. If congestion and sinus problems are making you miserable, there's a cheap, easy remedy — nasal irrigation.

This technique gently rinses out your nasal passages to get rid of any viruses, bacteria, pollen, allergens, dust, or mucus lurking there. Studies found that people who use nasal irrigation have fewer, less severe symptoms, and don't need antibiotics as often. If you want to try it, here's what you'll need.

- **A neti pot or bulb syringe.** You can find them both at most drugstores. Neti pots resemble Aladdin's magic lamp or a teapot, and a bulb syringe is a hollow tube with a squeezable bulb at one end.

- **Distilled or sterilized water.** Do not use tap water unless you bring it to a rolling boil for three minutes and let it cool. Otherwise it might contain a rare amoeba called *Naegleria fowleri*. It's completely harmless if swallowed, but if it gets in your nose it can travel up to your brain and cause a fatal infection.

- **Salt.** Try to use canning or picking salt, since table salt often contains additives that can irritate your nasal passages. If table salt is your only option, make sure to use the non-iodized kind.

▸ **Baking soda.** This buffers the salt to soothe your sinuses.

Mix one-half teaspoon salt and one-quarter teaspoon baking soda with one cup of water. Pour this mixture into your neti pot, or suction into the bulb syringe. Tilt your head sideways over a sink, and slowly pour or squeeze about half the mixture into one nostril so it runs out the other nostril. Turn your head to the other side, and pour the remaining mixture into the other nostril. Gently blow your nose after the water has drained out.

When you are finished, clean the neti pot or syringe with steril-ized water and let dry thoroughly. Any water left could harbor bacteria or other irritants.

Take note — rinsing daily for more than a year may actually make you more prone to sinus infections, possibly by washing away too much protective mucus.

Water — one natural sinusitis solution. It's essential to good health, involved in making every system in your body work properly. But water is also a surprising remedy for inflamed and painful sinuses. Check out these four ways simple water can make you feel better.

▸ **Get steamed up.** Lean over a bowl of hot — not boiling — water, cover your head with a towel to trap the steam, and inhale for 10 minutes. Do this up to four times a day. You can also use a sink full of water or simply breathe in the steam from a cup of hot water. For an extra boost, consider adding pine oil, eucalyptus, or menthol to the water.

▸ **Drink more.** Fluids, especially water, help lubricate swollen mucous membranes. Staying hydrated will thin and loosen the hardened mucus blocking your sinuses so it can drain away properly. Aim for at least six glasses a day.

▶ **Care for your air.** Even clean air can irritate sensitive sinuses, especially in winter months when it is particularly dry. Use a humidifier in your home to put moisture back into the air and make it easier to breathe.

▶ **Apply a compress.** Some people get relief by placing warm, water-soaked cloths directly over their sinuses.

Brew sinus-soothing teas from your spice rack. When you're sick, there's nothing better than a hot cup of tea. The warm liquid soothes your throat and the steam can help break up congestion. But if you need a little extra relief, ditch the tea bags and take advantage of the remedies hidden in your pantry. These teas made from spices could be just what you need to soothe your sinusitis.

▶ Peppermint tea is a powerful, old-fashioned remedy for a stuffy nose. That's because peppermint leaves contain a compound called menthol. When you get a whiff, the vapors react with the cold receptors in your nose and make you feel like you're breathing in more cool air. This reduces that uncomfortable stuffed-up feeling and makes you feel as if you have taken a decongestant pill — even though you haven't.

To make a cup, add one to two tablespoons of fresh peppermint leaves or two to three teaspoons of dried peppermint leaves to a cup of freshly boiled water. Let this steep for 10 minutes, taking a few sniffs of the steam while you wait. Add sweetener, if needed, and slowly sip the tea while it works its magic on your poor nose. You may be surprised at how much better you feel.

▶ Fennel and anise both contain anti-inflammatory compounds that can help clear your sinuses. To make them into tea, crush one teaspoon of fennel seeds or one-and-a-half teaspoons of anise seeds with a mortar and pestle. Add to a cup of boiling water, and let steep for 10 to 15 minutes. Strain through a fine sieve or coffee filter, and enjoy.

▸ Sage tea is one great way to soothe a sore throat, so if you're dealing with a bad postnasal drip, give it a try. Add a teaspoon of ground sage to a cup of boiling water and let it steep for about 15 minutes.

Rx Alert

Hold the meds! OTC sinus remedies a bust

When you've been wrestling with sinus pain, over-the-counter medicines seem so tempting. Watch out, though. You may breathe easier for a while, but a few hours later your symptoms will come back with a vengeance. That's because those drugs might actually be making your sinusitis worse.

Decongestants can increase inflammation, and research suggests they don't help treat sinusitis anyway. Many allergy and cold medicines contain antihistamines, which just dry up your mucus so it can't drain out.

Skin cancer

Every month you shed your skin. Fortunately it doesn't peel off all at once, but, little by little, you're constantly growing a whole new hide. Old cells die and slough off, while new ones form to replace them. The cells reproduce when they are needed, and stay where they are supposed to. It's a very orderly process.

At least it is until something triggers a skin cell to go rogue.

Think of it like this. You have stem cells in your skin that are a bit like a sourdough starter. When you're out of bread, you can just take a piece off and bake a fresh loaf. Now imagine that starter growing out of control and baking bread by itself. Instead of having loaves only when and where you need them, you wind up with an endless supply of "abnormal" bread.

That's what happens when you get skin cancer. Damage from ultraviolet (UV) radiation causes your stem cells to mutate, and they begin growing cancerous cells where normal skin cells should be.

And because everybody gets a dose of UV radiation when they step into the sun, skin cancer is the most widespread cancer in the United States. One out of every five Americans will develop it at some point in their lives.

Triple threat: the most common types of skin cancer. Basal cell carcinoma and squamous cell carcinoma make up almost 99 percent of all skin cancers. These are usually found in places on your body that get a lot of sun, like your arms, hands, face, and neck. Both types grow slowly and are rarely life-threatening, unless left untreated.

Melanoma is much rarer, but much more dangerous. Despite only making up 1 percent of new skin cancers, it is by far the most deadly. It starts in the lower layers of your skin and can spread easily throughout your body.

Check and check again to catch cancer early. A cancer diagnosis is always frightening, but there's a silver lining with skin cancer — it's easy to treat, as long as it's caught early.

Diagnosing your moles with smartphone apps or online medical services may seem like a great way to save some time and money, but the consequences could be deadly. Researchers discovered these services are prone to misdiagnoses. In one study, a top smartphone app incorrectly classified 30 percent of melanomas as benign.

You should examine yourself once a month, looking for warning signs. And don't neglect areas like your palms, under your fingernails, on your eyelids, and between your toes. If you have trouble with those hard-to-see spots, like your scalp or back, ask a loved one for help.

When you're on the hunt for suspicious moles, remember your ABCDEs. These are warning signs of melanoma.

- **Asymmetry.** The shape of one half doesn't match the other.

- **Border.** The edges are jagged or scalloped.

- **Color.** It's made up of a variety of colors.

▶ **Diameter.** The mole is larger than a pencil eraser.

▶ **Evolving.** The size, color, or shape changes.

See your doctor immediately if you have any of these symptoms, or sores that are slow to heal.

Are you at risk? Sun damage accumulates over time, so your risk of skin cancer gets higher every year. And while anyone can develop this potentially deadly condition, some people have to be more careful. If you sunburn easily or have fair skin, red hair, or even a family member with red hair, you might be extra sensitive to sunlight. If you've already had skin cancer, you have a good chance of getting it again.

The only way to completely avoid UV radiation is to never go outside. But who wants to live their whole life in the dark? Here are a few more practical ways you can cut your risk of skin cancer.

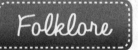 **Resveratrol supplements not worth the cash**

Have you heard it through the grapevine? Resveratrol can fight skin cancer. In numerous studies, this natural antioxidant, found in red grapes, prevented the kind of DNA damage from UVB light known to trigger cancer.

But if you're eating grapes by the bunch or taking resveratrol supplements, there's a problem — your body processes it so quickly you're not really getting any health benefits. Instead, researchers are turning to topical creams that put resveratrol right on your skin. Some products are on the market, but their effectiveness is still mostly unproven.

7 sun-sational tips block skin cancer

Ward off UV rays with your wardrobe. What you wear matters, especially when it comes to stopping the sun. UV rays can get through your clothes, so even when you're covered from head to toe, you're not really covered. Here's how to dress for skin cancer success.

▸ Choose dark, intense colors. Deeper, darker dyes give you more protection from the sun. Choose a dark blue shirt, for instance, over a light yellow one.

▸ Look for heavy, tightly woven fabrics. Hold your clothing up to the sun. If you can see sunlight shining through, it isn't going to protect you.

▸ Seek out UPF-rated clothing. Ultraviolet Protection Factor measures how much UV radiation can pass through your clothes. A 15 rating is good; 50 or higher is excellent. Usually clothing with this rating is treated with a chemical sunblock and uses fabric weave and colors that are most protective.

Caffeine fiends rejoice — your morning coffee has some serious perks. If you're a coffee drinker, you know the day doesn't really begin until you have that first sip. But what you probably don't know is your morning routine could be protecting your skin.

A recent review of seven observational studies shows people who regularly drink caffeinated coffee are less likely to get skin cancer than non-coffee drinkers or those who go with decaf. And the more you drink, the better. People who downed four or more cups of caffeinated coffee daily lowered their risk of melanoma by 20 percent compared to people who avoided coffee, according to a recent study published in the *Journal of the National Cancer Institute*.

The key to coffee's cancer-fighting prowess is the caffeine. It blocks UV rays from damaging your skin, just like sunscreen. Even better, it actually causes cancerous cells to die. Now, coffee shouldn't replace sunscreen or smart sun habits, but it's nice to know your morning joe comes with benefits.

Spice up your life to thwart skin cancer. People have always searched for ways to make their food tastier. Thousands of years ago they turned to turmeric. And while this spice is still popular in curries today, researchers are just beginning to scratch the surface of its exciting health benefits.

Turmeric's distinct yellow color is behind its cancer-fighting powers, thanks to a natural chemical called curcumin.

It works a lot like an email spam filter. Your cells are constantly sending messages back and forth. Most are helpful, but some are like computer viruses, actually causing cancerous cells to form. Curcumin blocks the harmful ones — the dangerous spam messages — and lets the rest through.

You can always take curcumin supplements, but there's evidence that suggests eating turmeric gives you more health benefits. If you're not sure you'll like it, test the waters by mixing a little bit into a homemade salad dressing or lightly seasoning some roasted veggies with it.

And whenever you eat turmeric, mix it with a bit of black pepper. It's a great flavor pairing and helps you absorb all the cancer-fighting nutrients.

Peppery turmeric vinaigrette

This salad dressing is a great way to add a splash of turmeric to your table. You'll need:

3 tblsp olive oil
1 tblsp apple cider vinegar
1 tblsp honey
2 tsp ground turmeric
1/2 tsp black pepper
a pinch of salt
a squeeze of lemon

Combine all the ingredients and whisk until everything is well combined. Drizzle over your favorite salad, or store covered in the refrigerator for later. It might separate, so mix well before serving.

Looking for a cancer-free future? Check your tea leaves.
Spanish explorer Ponce de Leon scoured the world for the mythical fountain of youth, but never found it. He might have been able to come close if he just had a few tea bags. Drinking a mug of green tea is almost as good as sipping from the legendary spring because it can fight off skin cancer and prevent your cells from aging.

Green tea is chock-full of natural plant chemicals called polyphenols that shield your skin from sun damage. Not only do they protect you from UV radiation, but they slow down wrinkles and make your skin look younger. It gets better — they also fight everything from heart disease and type 2 diabetes to flu and bad breath.

If you want to harness all of green tea's super powers, brew up a couple of steaming cups of this pleasant beverage every day. Just talk to your doctor before taking green tea supplements because they can cause severe liver damage.

Chocolate — the delicious secret that saves your skin. The magic is in natural chemicals found in cocoa beans, called flavanols. These fight off damaging free radicals and inflammation, and protect your skin from harmful UV rays, reducing your risk of skin cancer.

While flavanols are present in most forms of chocolate, they are highest in dark chocolate. But even so, a lot of the beneficial flavanols are lost during processing. To make matters worse, you won't find flavanols listed anywhere on labels.

- Lavado, sometimes called "unfermented cocoa," contains the most flavanols because it undergoes the least processing. The cacao beans are simply washed, dried, then ground. Look for this type of cocoa powder in health food stores or on the internet.

- Natural, or "non-alkalized," cocoa powder is made by fermenting the beans for several days, which destroys some of their flavanols. The cocoa powder sold in supermarkets is often natural cocoa.

- Dutch cocoa is the worst. Not only are the beans fermented, but they're also treated with an alkali solution to make the cocoa less acidic. All this processing removes up to 90 percent of its flavanols. Check ingredient lists for words like "alkalized," "European style," or "Dutched."

"B" on the lookout for this cancer-fighting supplement. "What's in a name? That which we call a rose by any other name would smell as sweet," Shakespeare wrote in his famous tale of star-crossed lovers. The Bard knew a lot about love, but he obviously never had to buy a vitamin B3 supplement. If you've ever seen the labels, you know there's a long list of complex options, all offering slightly different benefits. So how do you choose the right one?

If you're worried about skin cancer, reach for a bottle that says nicotinamide or niacinamide. This is the active form of niacin, a type of vitamin B3 found naturally in foods like meat, fish, and peanuts, and often added to cereals. However, you can only get trace amounts of nicotinamide from food.

A yearlong study showed that people with a history of skin cancer, who took 1,000 milligrams of nicotinamide a day, dramatically lowered their risk of new lesions. Researchers think the supplement actually repairs cell damage caused by UV radiation, preventing cancerous cells from forming.

Be careful not to overdo your nicotinamide supplements, however. They won't cause flushing, headaches, and low blood pressure like niacin, but they might cause liver damage if you take more than 3 grams a day. More than 2 grams a day can also decrease your insulin sensitivity. So if you're at risk for diabetes, ask your doctor before trying a high-dose supplement.

Boost omega-3 and safeguard your skin. Most people can't stand anchovies on pizza. But if they only knew what they were missing.

No, not just a tangy, salty treat, but a heaping helping of omega-3 fatty acids that protect you from skin cancer.

Still not sold on anchovies? Don't worry — other fish like salmon, mackerel, and trout are good sources, as well as walnuts, flaxseed, and fortified eggs.

Omega-3 fatty acids work by creating a buffer zone for your cells. They're one of the first targets for cancer-causing free radicals, so they take the damage instead of other parts of your body. And they help reduce inflammation and increase your resistance to UV rays, which helps prevent cancerous spots from forming.

Shoot for about 4 grams of omega-3 fatty acids a day to reap all the skin-saving benefits. You can get half that from a 3-ounce serving of salmon. If you're not a fish fan, consider supplements.

Warning

The tart truth: grapefruit linked to skin cancer

There are two things you should never do right after drinking grapefruit juice — brush your teeth and go out into the sun. One will leave a bad taste in your mouth, but the other raises your risk of melanoma.

Researchers discovered people who had citrus, especially grapefruit, every day had a 36 percent higher risk of malignant melanoma compared to those who enjoyed citrus only twice a week. It's because citrus fruits contain compounds called psoralens that increase your sensitivity to UV rays.

This doesn't mean you should stop eating citrus altogether. Just be extra careful with sun exposure.

Are you making these 4 deadly sunscreen mistakes?

You're not doing everything you can to stop skin cancer unless you're wearing sunscreen. But only 14 percent of men and 30 percent of women wear it regularly. And even if you are putting it on, you might not be as protected as you think. Don't fall for these dangerous sunscreen mistakes.

Mistake 1: You spend big bucks on a high-SPF sunscreen.
Most people look at one thing when they're buying sunscreen — the SPF, or sun protection factor. They think the higher this number, the more shielding they get. And while there's some truth to that, the differences aren't very big.

Every SPF number reflects a percentage of protection. For instance, SPF 15 blocks 93 percent of UVB rays, while SPF 30 blocks 97 percent, and SPF 50 blocks 98 percent. The differences become smaller as the numbers get bigger, so there's no real advantage in paying for ultra-high SPF sunscreens.

Mistake 2: You apply and forget about it. It doesn't matter how high the SPF is, sunscreen won't last all day. Reapply it every two hours — more frequently if you're sweating or splashing around in the water.

Mistake 3: You don't cover all your bases. If you're not wearing a broad-spectrum sunscreen, you're only stopping half the UV rays that cause skin damage. There are two types you need to worry about:

  ▶ UVB rays damage the top layers of your skin, causing sunburns.

▶ UVA rays penetrate deep into your skin and are tougher to block, getting to your skin even on cloudy days.

Mistake 4: You use too little, too late. Sunscreen takes time to start working. If you put it on when you're already outside, it's too late. You need to apply it 30 minutes before you step into the sun. And don't skimp. You need a golf-ball size amount to cover your whole body.

Don't miss your daily dose of vitamin D

New!

There's a reason they call vitamin D the sunshine vitamin. Your skin creates it just by soaking up sunlight.

But here's the dilemma. When you put on sunscreen, you not only protect your skin from the sun's harmful rays, you also block your ability to make all the vitamin D your body needs.

Now researchers have developed a new sunscreen to change that. Their product, called Solar D, carries an SPF of 30 or 50, yet still allows your body to make vitamin D. Visit the Solar D website at *solar-d.com* for more information.

Sleep apnea

Are you one of the 18 million Americans suffering from sleep apnea? If so, you're in historic company. Researchers suspect that plump, thick-waisted Queen Victoria had it, too. Her raucous snores rocked the British realm back in the day. And on this side of the pond, Franklin Roosevelt's rip-roaring snoring rattled the White House rafters on a regular basis. In fact, sleep apnea could have been a contributing factor to his death in 1945.

Wake up, little Susie, wake up. And pay attention. This sleep apnea is serious stuff.

Raise-the-roof snoring, gasping for breath during the night, and sleepiness during the day are all symptoms of obstructive sleep apnea (OSA). When you have OSA, the muscles in the back of your throat relax when you go to sleep, allowing your tongue to fall backwards and block off your airway. The result? You stop breathing. "Apnea" refers to this pause in your breathing that lasts at least 10 seconds. These pauses can happen a few times an hour, or as often as 100 times a night.

And snoring is not even the worst part. OSA opens the door for serious complications like high blood pressure, diabetes, heart attack, depression, and stroke. It's also been linked with hearing loss, memory problems, and loss of brain power at an earlier age than expected.

But just because you're a world-class snorer doesn't mean you have OSA. In fact, most people who snore don't. Keep one eye open for these warning signs — just in case.

▸ You're obese. About two-thirds of people diagnosed with OSA are overweight.

▸ You have a family history of snoring.

▸ You have a large neck. That's 17 inches or more for men and at least 16 inches for women.

▸ You have a large tongue, large tonsils, or a small jaw.

Already diagnosed with OSA? Read on to learn about some helpful ways you — and your spouse — can get back to enjoying a good night's sleep.

4 all-natural ways to defeat sleep apnea

Catch a few ZZZs with the catch of the day. What's the special tonight? Salmon, rainbow trout, sardines? Take your pick. All three contain an omega-3 fatty acid, called docosahexaenoic acid — DHA for short.

A major study published in the *Journal of Clinical Sleep Medicine* reports a strong relationship between the amount of DHA in your blood and how severe your sleep apnea is. The fatty acid not only impacts how hormones affect your circadian clock — your natural sleep-wake cycle — but could also affect nerves and muscles in your breathing passages.

"The brain and the body are deficient in the machinery to make DHA," says Fernando Gomez-Pinilla, a UCLA professor of neurosurgery. "It has to come through our diet."

That means stock up on wild salmon — farm-raised lacks the DHA punch. Two 4-ounce servings a week should do it. Or try a fish oil supplement, especially one high in DHA. When it comes to omega-3 fatty acids, it's actually safe, and healthy, to sleep with the fishes.

Sesame-ginger salmon

4 4-ounce salmon filets
1/4 cup peanut oil
1/2 tsp sesame oil
2 tblsp low-sodium soy sauce
2 tblsp balsamic vinegar
1 1/2 tsp brown sugar
1 garlic clove, minced
3/4 tsp ground ginger
1/2 tsp crushed red pepper flakes

Combine all marinade ingredients. Place salmon in a resealable plastic bag, and pour marinade in. Close bag and refrigerate for 4 to 6 hours, turning occasionally to coat fish.

Spray grill rack with nonstick cooking spray and preheat grill. Remove salmon from marinade and grill until fish flakes with a fork, turning halfway through cooking.

Try this simple formula to determine how long to grill or broil a fish.

1. Measure the piece of fish at its thickest point.

2. Cook it 10 minutes per inch for the first inch, five minutes on each side.

3. Add only one more minute per side for an additional inch, then test it.

Shed some pounds for sound sleep. You've probably heard that weight loss helps with chronic conditions like heart disease, diabetes, and cancer. Now you can add obstructive sleep apnea (OSA) to the list.

If you're overweight, you may have extra tissue in the back of your throat that blocks the air flow to your lungs while you sleep, causing your tiresome — and even dangerous — sleep apnea symptoms. Losing weight helps correct that.

And a little loss goes a long way. According to the Adult Obstructive Sleep Apnea Task Force of the American Academy of Sleep Medicine, dropping just 10 percent of your body weight can significantly improve your OSA. Losing a little more can even cure it.

A study published by the Perelman School of Medicine at the University of Pennsylvania agrees. "If you're overweight and often feel tired," says researcher Isaac Perron, "you may not need to lose all the weight to improve sleep." As you adjust your diet to improve your sleep apnea, you'll feel more awake and alert during the day, motivating you to continue your new, healthier lifestyle.

A trio of veggies means heart-healthy sleep. Peppers, spinach, broccoli. Sleep apnea superheroes.

All three contain a heaping helping of vitamins C and E, powerful antioxidants that can protect you from endothelial dysfunction. That's a fancy name for a condition linked to sleep apnea, where your blood vessels don't relax and contract like they're supposed to. It can lead to some pretty serious problems, including heart disease and stroke.

So protect your heart from the scary side effects of sleep apnea with delicious foods — and enjoy those sweet dreams.

Dance your way to dreamland? You bet, say sleep experts. Studies prove that about 40 minutes of dancing or other moderate aerobic exercise four times a week — along with some weight training twice a week — will help relieve your obstructive sleep apnea symptoms.

Researchers aren't really sure why exercise works. They think it improves muscle tone, but it could also help with vein and artery problems that spring up with OSA.

And it doesn't even seem to matter if you lose weight as you amp up your exercise program. Drop the pounds or not, you'll still reap the benefits of better quality sleep at night, less sleepiness during the day.

Go mask-free with these sleep solutions

CPAP therapy — short for continuous positive airway pressure — is still the king of the hill when it comes to treating obstructive sleep apnea (OSA). But if it's not right for you, here are some alternatives that might do the trick.

Disposable nasal valves. These stick to your nostrils like small, round bandages and create pressure when you exhale, which in turn keeps your airway open. How effective are they? Researchers have seen a 40 percent improvement in mild and moderate cases of OSA. While they only cost a couple of dollars each, you do have to replace them every night, so your investment definitely adds up. In addition, you'll need a doctor's prescription.

Mandibular advancement device (MAD). Up to 90 percent effective in treating OSA, these custom-made mouth guards work by pushing your jaw forward, which keeps your tongue from falling back into your airway and blocking your airflow. MADs can be pricey, costing upwards of $2,200, but many are covered by health insurance or Medicare. Studies suggest MADs also help reduce your blood pressure just as well as CPAP machines.

Hypoglossal nerve stimulator (HGNS). Now there's a mouthful. This surgically implanted device works like a pacemaker for sleep. An electrode in your chest senses when you start to inhale. Then another electrode, placed in your throat, stimulates your tongue to tighten, which keeps it from blocking your airway. The third part of the device is the generator — the power source — that's inserted just below your collarbone.

Doctors say this pacemaker is shown to improve OSA symptoms by about 70 percent. But it's not recommended for people who are extremely overweight or who suffer from severe sleep apnea.

End slumber troubles with easy snore stoppers

Not everyone who snores has sleep apnea. But anyone who snores may find themselves face to face with an angry, sleepy spouse by dawn's early light. Put a stop to your snoring once and for all with these five simple suggestions.

Try mouth and tongue exercises. A Brazilian study showed that snorers who practiced tongue exercises snored 36 percent less, and turned down the volume on their snoring by a whopping 59 percent.

Here's one to try. Push the tip of your tongue against the roof of your mouth, then slide it backwards. Repeat 20 times every day.

Use pillows to raise your chest. Propping yourself up about 45 degrees means less pressure on your airway and less snoring. A steady flow of oxygen will cut your risk of dangerously irregular heart rhythms, too.

Tape up your nose. With age, the tip of your nose may begin to droop. Figures, right? And this droop can block your nasal passages, making it harder for you to breathe. Try a simple test. Push the tip of your nose up. If this makes it easier for you to breathe, cut a few inches of 1/2-inch-wide medical tape. Gently lift the tip of your nose and run the tape from the tip, up the bridge of your nose to between your eyes. Be careful not to block your airway.

It's a fact — 90 million Americans, both men and women, snore. If you're one of them, your troubles could be more serious than disturbing your spouse's slumber. Snoring is linked to health issues like type 2 diabetes, high blood pressure, and memory problems. Don't put off calling your doctor. You snooze, you lose.

Wear compression socks. Researchers in Canada found that wearing below-the-knee compression stockings only during the day reduced sleep apnea symptoms at night. The stockings work by squeezing the lower legs to keep your blood circulating. This stops the buildup of fluid in your neck that contributes to snoring.

Make some music. Try an oboe, a bassoon, or an English horn. Studies found that playing one of these double-reed wind instruments helped control snoring by strengthening upper respiratory system muscles. Singing works, too. British researchers discovered semiprofessional singers enjoyed better sleep than non-singers — they snored less and not as loudly.

Asleep at the wheel? How you can steer clear of drowsy driving accidents

Getting behind the wheel when you haven't had a good night's sleep is dangerous — for you and everyone else on the road, yet more than half of all drivers have done it. No one plans to nod off while driving, but it's more likely to happen if you slept less than six hours the night before, or if you snore.

The National Sleep Foundation says the following are signs you, or the driver in your car, need to stop and take a rest.

▶ blurry vision, frequent blinking, or drooping eyelids

▶ trouble keeping your head up

▶ yawning

▶ feeling as if you're driving in a trance

▶ missing exits or traffic signs

▶ drifting from your lane, tailgating, or hitting a shoulder rumble strip

▶ restlessness or irritability

So now that you know the warning signs of fatigue — you must heed them. Here's what to do to make sure you don't fall asleep at the wheel.

Bring a friend. You're more likely to experience a drowsy driving crash if you're traveling alone. Have someone else in the car with you to help you stay awake and to watch for signs of fatigue.

Stop driving. Pull off as soon as possible to a rest area, restaurant, or hotel.

Take a nap. You only need to sleep for 15 to 20 minutes. More than that and you'll be too groggy to drive right away.

Pop in some gum. Need a reason to carry a pack of gum in your car? It could save your life. Research shows chewing gum can make you more alert. While the sugarless variety is best for your teeth, minty or cinnamon-flavored will really pep you up. A West Virginia study found that people who drove a long time felt more alert when the scent of cinnamon or peppermint was in the air.

Consume some caffeine. It takes about 30 minutes for caffeine to enter your bloodstream, so plan ahead. Remember, you can get an eye-popping dose from soft drinks, tea, and energy drinks. One cup of coffee can have as much as 200 milligrams of caffeine.

In addition, be careful about taking allergy and pain medications, tranquilizers, alcohol, and sleep aids. They can stay in your system far longer than you might think and can make you drowsy even the next day.

Thinning hair

Thick, shiny hair — the stuff legends are made of. It brought Rapunzel her handsome prince, protected Lady Godiva's secrets, and gave Samson his epic strength. You spend hours curling it, dying it, brushing it. But lately you're spending lots of time counting it, as more strands show up in your comb. What's behind this upsetting change? And how can you head it off?

Experts at the American Academy of Dermatology say your hair woes can be triggered by factors such as weight loss, stress, hormones, haircare products, or even your favorite hairstyle. You have about 100,000 hairs on your head, so losing an average of 50 to 100 strands a day is no big deal — until you notice lots of hair in the shower drain or bald patches on your scalp.

So what else could be causing your tress distress?

Genetics. The most common cause is hereditary thinning or baldness. Known in the medical world as androgenetic alopecia, it affects about 80 million men and women in the U.S. Other hair-nabbing conditions include an autoimmune disease called alopecia areata, and cicatricial alopecia, a disorder that destroys hair follicles.

Disease. About 30 ailments, including thyroid disease and anemia, can result in hair loss. So can a high fever, a severe infection, or even the flu.

Nutrition. Too much vitamin A, taken either through supplements or medicines, can make you lose your hair. Too little protein in your diet — like eggs, meat, or fish — and not enough iron — the mineral found in spinach, clams, and pumpkin seeds — will also thin your locks.

Hair loss, in a nutshell

Nuts can be a healthy addition to your diet — as long as you don't overdo it.

Take Brazil nuts, for example. They're famous for their abundance of selenium, a trace mineral that provides good-for-you antioxidants. Get too much selenium in your system, though, and you might find yourself facing hair-raising symptoms like fatigue, stomach upset, and — you guessed it — hair loss.

An ounce of Brazil nuts, about six to eight of the crunchy kernels, contains 544 micrograms (mcg) of selenium. But the National Institutes of Health recommends a daily selenium dose of just 55 mcg, and no more than 400 mcg. Makes you reconsider that can of mixed nuts, doesn't it?

And while it's true that Brazil nuts have the highest selenium content out there, you can find the mineral in other foods like tuna, clams, and turkey. Bottom line, when it comes to selenium, a little bit goes a long, long way.

Medications. Prescription drugs like blood thinners could be to blame. Other culprits include medicines that treat your high blood pressure, depression, gout, or heart problems. Talk to your doctor if you have concerns.

Looking for some treatments to challenge your hair loss? Well, heads up. Here are three ways to make every day a great hair day.

3 hair 'do's' for thicker tresses

Protein — perfect for healthy hair repair. Need a little tress relief? You could just chow down on a natural beauty staple. For growing stronger, thicker hair, there's nothing like a good egg. It really is all it's cracked up to be.

Protein is essential for thick, healthy hair, and as a source of protein, it's hard to beat an egg. The Food and Nutrition Board of the Institute of Medicine says women need 46 grams (g) of protein a day and men 56 g. Just one large egg gives you six of those grams. And eggs also provide you with iron, a mineral important for maintaining your shiny mane.

If you're concerned about extra fat and cholesterol, stick to the egg white. You'll miss out on the iron, but you'll still get lots of follicle-fortifying nutrition — without the extra calories.

Essential therapy for hair loss. Try this root stimulator made from fragrant essential oils, and be ready to get out your comb.

Lavender essential oil, combined with cedarwood, thyme, and rosemary oils, has been shown to help regrow hair — if your hair loss is due to alopecia areata, an autoimmune disease where your body's immune system attacks your hair follicles. In one study, more than half of the people treated with this aromatic mixture reported positive results after seven months.

Want to give it a try? You can find essential oils at herb shops, health food stores, and drugstores. Here's the formula.

Essential oils:

▸ 3 drops lavender oil (*Lavandula agustifolia*)

▸ 3 drops rosemary oil (*Rosmarinus officinalis*)

▸ 2 drops cedarwood oil (*Cedrus atlantica*)

▸ 2 drops thyme oil (*Thyme vulgaris*)

Carrier oils:

▸ 1/2 teaspoon jojoba oil   ▸ 4 teaspoons grapeseed oil

To use, blend the oils together. Massage into your scalp for two minutes each night. Wrap your head in a warm towel to help your skin absorb the oils.

For thicker hair, choose green cuisine. When it comes to getting the right nutrients for luxuriant, shiny hair, you can't beat the green giant, turnip greens. They are absolutely chock-full of lock-loving vitamins.

▸ Take vitamin A, for instance. Just one cup of cooked turnip greens supplies more than twice your recommended dietary allowance (RDA) of vitamin A, the nutrient you need to produce sebum, a natural hair moisturizer.

▸ And that same cup of turnip greens also provides two-thirds of your RDA of vitamin C, which your body uses to make collagen — a type of protein that forms connective tissue inside your hair follicles.

▸ Since low iron is a common cause of hair loss, you'll want to pump up your levels. Vitamin C boosts your ability to absorb iron, so eat foods rich in both. Lucky for you, turnip greens fit the bill.

These leafy greens also contain whopping levels of vitamin K, so if you are taking blood thinners, talk to your doctor before including this vegetable in your diet.

Take care of your fragile hair

Every time you gel, spray, tease, or highlight, you're breaking delicate strands of hair and inching your way further down the road to hair loss. Dermatologist Amy McMichael offers these suggestions for better hair care.

Stop damaging practices. Hot rollers, curling irons, harsh chemicals, hot oil treatments, tight braids — all these can be stressful to your scalp. If you don't correct the damage they do before scarring occurs, hair loss can be permanent, McMichael says.

Minimize breakage with a little pampering. Use moisturizing shampoos and conditioners. And McMichael suggests getting your hair trimmed every six to eight weeks. Stylists are often the first to notice signs of hair loss.

Trust your hair to an expert. If you use two or more hair treatments — such as color and a perm — see a qualified hair stylist, McMichael advises. Don't try to do it yourself. Although some people manage it without harmful effects, she says most people aren't so lucky.

A laser light could rouse your scalp

New!

Shock your follicles back into growth mode with a treatment straight out of the Jetsons. It's called low-level laser therapy (LLLT), and it was given the nod of approval by the FDA in 2011.

Caps, headbands, helmets, combs — these are all pricey devices that promise lush tresses through laser treatments. But can they really wake up your lethargic locks?

Proponents of LLLT say yes. While LLLT doesn't promise to bring dead follicles back to life, it can stimulate those that have slowed down production, so you see thicker, fuller hair.

Studies have shown — and satisfied customers report — that LLLT is a safe and effective treatment for androgenetic and chemotherapy-induced alopecia, as well as alopecia areata. George Jetson would be pleased.

Vision loss

You use them to locate your phone every morning, to sort through your medication, and to navigate the open road. Your eyes are a precious part of your life. Unfortunately, aging eyes can make everyday tasks — even reading this page — more difficult. So why, exactly, do you have to hold the newspaper at arms length in order to read the morning headlines?

Just like the rest of your body, your eyes change over time. During your early to mid-40s, your sharp vision may start to get a little fuzzy. This is because, as you get older, the lenses in your eyes become thicker, harder, and less elastic. On top of that, the muscles that control your lenses begin to weaken.
The result is your eyes cannot focus like they used to. This is a frustrating, but normal condition called presbyopia.

Don't let aging eyes steal your vision. Weaker eyes may be normal, but some common eye conditions can spell a bigger problem.

▸ **Age-related macular degeneration (AMD).** If you're age 50 or older, you may be at risk for this eye disease. AMD means you have damage to the macula, the most sensitive part of the retina, located on the back of your eyeball. When your macula is impaired, things that are straight ahead may seem blurry. Imagine trying to drive with a dark spot where the traffic light is supposed to be. Yikes.

▸ **Cataracts.** The lens of your eye, made of mostly protein and water, is supposed to be clear. When working normally, it helps focus light on the back of your eyeball. As you age, bits of protein start clumping together, and form cloudy areas in the lens called cataracts. These make you feel like you're gazing through a foggy window. Experts estimate that, by age 80, more than half of all Americans either have a cataract or have had one surgically removed.

▶ **Glaucoma.** This disease, most common in folks over age 60, brings new meaning to the phrase "tunnel vision." When fluid within your eye cannot flow in and out properly, it builds up, and creates a dangerous amount of pressure inside your eyeball — like a balloon filled with too much air. If this pressure damages your optic nerve, visual info doesn't make it from your retina to your brain. Left untreated, you could slowly lose your peripheral vision, and end up viewing the world through a dark tunnel.

Steer clear of habits that hurt your eyes. Your body doesn't grow old overnight. Chemical "crooks" called free radicals do the dirty work over time. These unstable molecules form when your body processes the oxygen you breathe. If you don't have enough antioxidants in your system to balance them, the free radicals will steal electrons from other molecules. This can cause a chain reaction of cell damage, called oxidation.

Scientists believe this domino effect plays a major role in aging, contributing to eye conditions such as cataracts, AMD, and glaucoma. Luckily, you can help fight free radicals by tweaking your lifestyle.

▶ Stop smoking to reduce your risk of AMD and cataracts.

▶ Defend your eyes with sunglasses that offer 100 percent protection from ultraviolet (UV) radiation — both UVA and UVB rays. Or look for a UV 400 sticker, which means the same thing.

▶ Power up on antioxidants by eating more fruits and veggies.

The good news is you have even more natural ways to battle the blur.

Vitamins and vision: it's time to get eye wise

The supplements you take to support your aging bones and eyes may not be as helpful as you think — and they could even be harmful.

- Too much calcium is linked to a higher risk of developing AMD, scientists recently reported in *JAMA Ophthalmology*. The danger appears greatest for older people who take more than 800 milligrams a day. Why? It's possible calcium particles in the retina attract proteins and fats which, over time, develop into deposits called drusen, an early sign of AMD.

- More than half of the top-selling eye supplements don't measure up to claims put on their labels. A landmark eye-disease study identified a specific vitamin formula that slows the development of AMD. But only four of the top 11 products contain those proven ingredients in the recommended doses. Despite that, all still claim to support and protect your vision.

Talk to your doctor before starting supplements, to get the nutrients you need.

Protect aging eyes with 6 tried-and-true tactics

Gobble up greens to prevent eye damage. I love kale — said no one, ever. Although you may not like leafy greens, your eyes crave them.

Swiss chard, kale, spinach, and collards are packed with lutein and zeaxanthin — two natural plant chemicals that go straight to your eyes to fight age-related vision loss. There they shield your eyes from light damage and free radicals. Lutein has also been known to reverse inflammation that can damage your baby blues.

Solid research shows this duo can slim down your chances of developing the three most common age-related eye problems.

▸ A recent study published in *JAMA Ophthalmology* took data from more than 100,000 people in the Nurses' Health Study and the Health Professionals Follow-up Study. Researchers found those who got the most lutein and zeaxanthin had about a 40 percent lower risk of advanced age-related macular degeneration, compared to those who got little of these phytochemicals.

▸ Eat plenty of foods high in these two nutrients, and you may reduce your need for cataract surgery. And University of Florida research confirms the more lutein and zeaxanthin you have in your eye tissues, the less likely you are to get cataracts in the first place.

▸ Just two servings of kale or collards a week dropped the risk of glaucoma by 57 percent in older African-American women, compared to those who ate the greens about once a month.

Combat cloudy vision with all-natural cataract preventers.
How many vitamin C-rich foods do you have in your kitchen
right now? Peppers? Oranges? Grapefruit? How about strawberries
or tomatoes? All of these will help you fight the leading cause of
blindness in the world — cataracts.

Vitamin C keeps your vision sharp by cracking down on
cataracts, reports the American Academy of Ophthalmology.
Folks who ate the most fruits and veggies high in this super
nutrient had a 19 percent lower risk of developing age-related
cataracts. And 10 years later, they were 33 percent less likely to
have their cataracts get worse.

"While we cannot totally avoid developing cataracts, we may
be able to delay their onset and keep them from worsening by
eating a diet rich in vitamin C," said study author Christopher
Hammond, M.D., professor of ophthalmology at King's
College London.

Walk your way to healthy sight. Your eyes may be doing more
than just taking in the beautiful scenery on your morning
march. As you work out your body, you're also keeping your
eyes in tiptop shape.

Can't believe simply
taking a brisk stroll
through the park
can fight aging eyes?
Check out the results
of a study recently pub-
lished in the journal
Ophthalmology. For 20
years, researchers moni-
tored the eye health of

Yoga's downward dog and forward bend poses leave some
people feeling recharged. But for
those with glaucoma, or at risk of
the disease, these head-down
positions are more distressing
than refreshing. Researchers out
of Columbia University Medical
Center say they are linked to a
rapid rise in eye pressure.

nearly 5,000 adults. In the end, they learned active folks had a 58 percent lower risk of vision loss compared to couch potatoes.

Other studies agree. Pulling on your tennis shoes may protect against the worst eye offenders — cataracts, glaucoma, and AMD.

Eat a heart-healthy diet to protect your peepers. Heap on the veggies, fruits, legumes, whole grains, fish, and nuts, and you've got one recipe for a health makeover. All these delicious foods are part of the Mediterranean diet, which is famous for helping your heart and reducing risk for diabetes, Alzheimer's disease, and certain cancers. Now, research shows this nutritious plan may also slow down AMD.

The study followed 2,525 participants in the AREDS (Age-Related Eye Disease Study). These people already had early stages of AMD, but those that stuck to a Mediterranean diet were 26 percent less likely to progress to advanced AMD over the next 13 years. It turns out taking your taste buds to the Mediterranean could boost your vision.

Go for grapes — they're a feast for your eyes. To improve the chances your eyes won't need glasses, contact lenses, surgery, drugs, or medicine of any kind as you get older, add grapes to your diet. They battle the damage that often leads to AMD.

Like a satellite picks up signals and converts them to an image on a TV screen, cells in your retina receive light signals that your brain sees as a picture. When people talk about AMD, they're really talking about injury to one small spot near the center of your retina, called the macula. It contains millions of light-sensitive cells that allow you to see what is directly in front of you. When these cells are damaged, oxidation is often to blame.

Surprisingly, grapes can counter this free radical damage. They contain antioxidants that protect healthy cells from harm, University of Miami researchers found.

"Adding grapes to the diet actually *preserved* retinal health in the presence of oxidative stress," said lead investigator Abigail S. Hackam, Ph.D., associate professor of ophthalmology at the Miller School of Medicine.

Although this was an animal study, researchers say these results add to previous evidence that grapes offer real benefits to your vision.

Safeguard your sight with a breakfast favorite. You don't have to be a morning person to jump-start your day with a vision-boosting breakfast. Swap that donut for a bowl of whole-grain cereal, and lower your risk of AMD, says a study published in the *American Journal of Clinical Nutrition*. Scientists think it's because cereal fiber helps steady your glucose levels, minimizing blood sugar spikes that can damage your eyes.

But whole-grain breakfast cereals contain so much more. They boast a natural helping of vitamins and minerals that also support your vision. And many are enriched with an extra dollop of these nutrients.

▸ **Zinc.** Did you know you can find this mineral in the part of your eye most affected by AMD? It works with a number of vitamins and antioxidants to protect against this sight-stealing condition. Women are encouraged to get 8 milligrams (mg) of zinc a day, men 11 mg.

▶ **B vitamins.** Whether it's a flake or a puff, most cereals are fortified with folate and vitamins B12 and B6. These nutrients lower levels of homocysteine, an amino acid linked to several eye diseases. A large study found that women who supplemented with these B vitamins reduced their risk of developing AMD.

▶ **Antioxidants.** Set your sights on vitamins A, C, and E to fight free radicals. Studies show this trio defends against age-related cataracts and macular degeneration.

Hocus-focus: cataract drops not ready for prime time

New!

Cure cataracts without surgery? It may someday be a real possibility, and all you'll need are special eye drops.

Scientists are exploring at least two compounds that seem to dissolve the protein clumps responsible for vision-stealing cataracts. And they've had some success on animals. But none have yet been approved by the Food and Drug Administration.

Weight control

"The only way to keep your health is to eat what you don't want, drink what you don't like, and do what you'd rather not," wrote Mark Twain. In other words, be miserable.

But it doesn't have to be that way. Suppose you could drop that four-letter word — diet — from your vocabulary for good, and replace it with a plan that would help you eat well and feel great? Sound too good to be true? It's not. Read on to find out how you can slim down and live a healthy life — once and for all.

Make good health your goal. Forget about squeezing into those skinny jeans. They weren't that comfortable anyway. Instead, focus on making lifestyle changes that result in a healthier you.

Take a few tips from the world's longest-living people. The highest concentrations of healthy centenarians in the world live tucked away in regions scientists call Blue Zones. And these zones are scattered all over the globe — in Greece, Japan, Italy, Costa Rica, and even the good old USA. What makes these folks more likely to live to be 100? Their healthy lifestyles.

In general, Blue Zoners share the following traits.

- They eat a plant-based diet with lots of beans — like fava beans, black beans, soybeans, and lentils — and very little meat.

- They make low-intensity exercise — walking, biking, swimming, and gardening — a part of their natural, daily routine.

▸ They build strong relationships with friends and family.

▸ They've found a purpose and meaning in life that inspires them to get out of bed every morning.

Just a few simple lifestyle choices like these can help you whittle your waist, and fight off serious conditions like cancer, diabetes, and heart disease.

Learn the basics of healthy living. Calories, portion control, BMI. Terms every dieter recognizes — and dreads. You'd like to forget about them, but don't. Instead, get to know them. Think of them as important tools to help you reach your goals.

What else will help? Choosing whole foods instead of processed. Eating less sugar and salt. Watching the kinds of fats you eat. Finding an exercise program you actually enjoy.

The bottom line — set realistic goals, make smart food choices, and adopt healthy habits that will stay with you for life.

So why "weight"? It's time to trade in your bathroom scale for a balanced life plan that can help you head off disease, peel away the pounds, and keep you fit and fabulous. Read on for some simple strategies designed to put you on the path to years and years of robust, vibrant health — maybe even 100 of them.

12 no-fail ways to stop dieting and lose the weight forever

Pump up the protein for a strong, slender you. The building blocks for healthy body tissues — like muscle, skin, and bone — are found in protein. So when you think about living a long, healthy life, consider this, protein is the one nutrient your body must have to stay strong as you age.

Sarcopenia is the gradual loss of muscle strength that naturally happens as you grow older. It can begin as early as age 40 and may lead to frailty and a higher risk of falls. Bye-bye, independence. Researchers at Tufts University found that a healthy diet of high-quality protein, along with some aerobic exercise and strength training, can help you hold onto your muscles.

Protein can also help peel off those extra pounds. High-protein foods signal your body that it's time to release some peptide YY (PYY), a hunger-squashing hormone that binds with receptors in your brain. These receptors decrease your appetite by making you feel full. And that makes it easier to walk away from those calorie-crammed snacks.

But be choosy when picking your proteins. Although animal products — like red and processed meats — can provide complete proteins, they are also linked with a higher risk of heart disease, colon cancer, and diabetes.

Avoid these risks by pumping up your menu with plant-based proteins, instead. To get you started, take a good look at lentils, the Biblical food that can be a modern saving grace. One cup packs a punch of almost 18 grams of protein, actually triggering your body to release PYY, so you eat less and feel full.

If that's not enough, studies show this powerhouse legume contains other nutrients that can help you lower your cholesterol, avoid cancer, dodge diabetes, and even protect your eyesight.

On the following page are seven more plant-based, protein-packed foods that practically force your body to lose weight. Why not give them a try?

Plant-based protein	Serving	Protein (grams)
Black-eyed peas, cooked	1 cup	13
Kidney beans, canned	1 cup	13
Quinoa, cooked	1 cup	8
Soymilk	1 cup	7
Pistachio nuts, dry-roasted	1/4 cup	6.5
Sunflower seeds, dry-roasted	1/4 cup	6
Oatmeal, cooked	1 cup	6

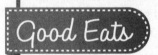 **Figure protein into your daily meal plan**

How much protein should you eat every day? Experts recommend about 7 grams for every 20 pounds of body weight. So if you weigh 140 pounds, figure around 49 grams of protein every day.

Watch out. Those protein grams add up quickly.

For example, start with a cup of low-fat, plain yogurt for breakfast. That's 14 grams of protein right off the bat. Your lunch menu could occasionally include a 4-ounce hamburger made from 90-percent lean beef. That's a whopping 28 grams of protein. Snack on a handful of almonds — 6 protein grams — and you're done for the day.

For a protein recommendation based on your weight, height, and age, plug your numbers into the online nutrition calculator at *nal.usda.gov/fnic/interactiveDRI*.

A flat belly can be yours with the right fat. When it comes to losing weight around your middle, it's often not how much you eat, but what you eat. And nothing will help you fight stubborn belly fat better than monounsaturated fats — MUFAs, for short.

Just how do MUFAs work this magic? One type, called oleic acid, releases a hunger-fighting super-substance in your small intestine that triggers a feeling of fullness — so you don't feel like snacking all the time. And recent studies show MUFAs also fire up a fat-burning process in your cells that keeps dangerous fat from building around your waist.

Surprise — simply "eating in moderation" won't help you lose weight, according to a University of Georgia study. Researchers found the more you like a food, the larger your "moderate" portion becomes. Instead, pull out your measuring cup and match your portion to the recommended serving size. You could save around 500 calories a day.

Here are five of the many delicious MUFA-rich foods that can help you achieve that slim waistline — olives, olive oil, avocados, nuts like almonds and pecans, and chocolate.

Wait. Chocolate?

That's right. An ounce of dark chocolate made with 70 to 85 percent cacao solids — check the label for this info — contains almost 4 grams of healthy fat. Just don't get carried away. This same ounce of sweet delight also adds 168 calories to your menu.

Want more good news? Not only will MUFAs help you stay slim and trim, anti-aging superfoods rich in monounsaturated fatty acids also keep your memory sharp and your heart healthy — maybe even into your 90s and beyond.

▶ Experts say MUFAs reduce your risk for heart disease by lowering your bad cholesterol — the LDL kind — while maintaining your good HDL cholesterol.

▶ MUFAs keep your brain healthy, too. During a four-year study of 6,000 women, researchers at Harvard University discovered the women who ate the most MUFAs scored higher on tests of brain function and memory than women who ate saturated fats — the kind found in red meat and butter.

Substituting MUFA-rich foods for those containing bad saturated fats is one easy way to keep your weight in check and your brain and heart set for a long, healthy life.

Stop the stress and lose the fat. "Stressed" spelled backwards is "desserts." And that's more than just a coincidence. How many times have you come home from a stressful day at work and grabbed a pint of ice cream from the freezer — almost before you take off your coat? Don't despair. You're not weak-willed or undisciplined. You're just made this way.

Whenever you feel stressed, your brain tells your adrenal glands to release cortisol, the "fight or flight" hormone. It's cortisol's job to tell your cells to replace the energy you used fighting or fleeing from whatever stressed you out — even if you didn't burn many calories. All this cortisol in your system can make you feel very hungry. And not for apples or celery sticks.

The power of chocolate — or pasta — is real. It works this way. Cortisol causes you to crave sweet, salty, and high-fat treats because those foods tip off the brain to release chemicals that make you feel less tense. And to make matters worse, this feel-good sensation is addicting, making you reach for ice cream — or chocolate or mac 'n cheese — whenever you're stressed.

Cortisol causes weight gain around your middle. Besides amping up your food cravings, cortisol makes your body store fat, especially visceral fat around your waist — the kind that can lead to heart problems and other chronic diseases.

Go from stressed out to slimmed down with these four suggestions.

> A messy kitchen is bad news for your waistline. In one study, women who spent time in a cluttered, chaotic kitchen — dirty dishes, ringing phone — ate twice as many cookies in just 10 minutes as those who were in a quiet, organized kitchen. Researchers say being in the disorderly kitchen led to feelings of stress — a significant cause of overeating.

▸ **Walk it off.** One of the best ways to wind down and let go of worries is to take a walk. There's a rhythm to it that's soothing, especially if you refuse to let your mind dwell on problems as you amble along. If you walk outside, you'll reap even more benefits. Scientists have found walking in a forest or park lowers levels of cortisol and boosts your immune function at the same time.

▸ **Get a good night's sleep.** The National Sleep Foundation recommends seven to nine hours of shut-eye every night for adults ages 18 to 64. Less than that could stress your body out and raise those cortisol levels.

▸ **Avoid caffeine.** Stimulants like caffeine can increase your stress levels — and your cortisol.

▸ **Eat your fruit and vegetables.** Enjoy lots of flavonoid-rich foods like apples, blueberries, and grapefruit that block cortisol production. A delicious way to lower your stress — and reduce your weight.

Waist measurement: inch your way to better health

Who Knew?

Your doctor may peg you as overweight or obese because your body mass index (BMI) is too high. Sorry Doc, wrong number.

Turns out you can have a normal BMI, but still carry extra fat around your middle. And that fat puts you at a higher risk for stroke and heart attack. On the other hand, a very muscular person — with little body fat — can have a high BMI. Confusing, isn't it?

Experts say a better way to measure your health is to check your waist circumference. Sneaky abdominal fat can't hide from a tape measure.

Keep in mind an ideal waist size for women is 32 inches or less, 37 inches or less for men. A waist measuring more than 35 inches for women — or 40 for men — raises your chances for heart disease, stroke, and even cancer.

So pull out that tape and measure your middle. Good health may be only inches away.

Peel off pounds with these carb favorites. Looking for a food that will control your hunger for hours and hours — and help you lose weight? Wouldn't it be great if an all-time favorite like pasta fit the bill? Surprise! It does.

Pasta, whole grains, and beans are just a few of the many foods containing resistant starch, a carbohydrate that "resists" digestion in your small intestine and moves straight to your colon. There, it acts as a prebiotic — a favorite food of the millions of good bacteria living in your colon. The bacteria ferment the resistant starch, forming short-chain fatty acids — like butyrate — that fuel the cells lining your colon. Short-chain fatty acids are the rock stars of your colon. They aid in controlling your appetite, regulating your blood sugar, and nurturing a healthy immune system.

And remember PYY — the hunger-crushing hormone that tells your brain your stomach's full? You can rev up your PYY by combining resistant starch and protein. You won't feel hungry, so you'll eat less. And your extra weight? Gone. Lickety-split.

Researchers say the average person eats about 4 grams of resistant starch daily, the amount in just half a cup of navy beans. But twice that would be much better.

To add more to your diet, chill out. When regular starches are cooked and then cooled, some of the starch changes into resistant starch. So if you refrigerate your spaghetti overnight, or make a cold potato into a little potato salad, you bump up its resistant starch about 1 percent.

Supercharge rice with this simple tip

Boost your resistant starch and cut calories with this easy way to cook rice. Add a teaspoon of coconut oil to your boiling water, pour in about one-half cup of rice, and let simmer for 40 minutes. Refrigerate the cooked rice for at least 12 hours. Then just warm it up and enjoy. That's all there is to it.

Researchers say this method of preparing rice raises its resistant starch level by 10 times. And it may even reduce the total calories by up to 60 percent.

Timing is everything when it comes to losing weight. Your body's internal clock is set to get your metabolism up and running first thing in the morning. With this in mind, researchers suggest you eat your meals early in the day to take advantage of your metabolism's prime time. Studies show it's a great way to reduce hunger swings — and even increase nighttime fat burning.

"We found that eating between 8 a.m. and 2 p.m. followed by an 18-hour daily fast kept appetite levels more even throughout the day, in comparison to eating between 8 a.m. and 8 p.m., which is what the average American does," said Courtney Peterson, Ph.D., associate professor in the Department of Nutrition Sciences at the University of Alabama, Birmingham.

But is 18 hours too long for you to go without a snack? Try this approach instead. Start with a healthy breakfast. Then eat most of your daily calories at lunch. Finally, enjoy a light dinner. In a 12-week study of 69 women, those who ate a larger lunch lost an average of three pounds more than the group who ate a big dinner.

And in a five-month study of 420 people, researchers found that those who ate an earlier lunch — before 3 p.m. — lost an average of five pounds more than those eating later. And the late-eaters lost weight at a much slower rate and had lower insulin sensitivity, a risk factor for diabetes.

Shakespeare probably wasn't concerned with his weight when he wrote, "Better three hours too soon than a minute too late." A diet guru ahead of his time? Maybe. But today's nutrition experts know the facts — when it comes to weight control, timing really is everything.

Pick plants to stem weight gain. Garfield creator Jim Davis wrote, "Vegetables are a must on a diet. I suggest carrot cake, zucchini bread, and pumpkin pie." You can be sure he'd approve of blueberry buckle and strawberry shortcake, too. Not great for weight control. But if you weed out all the bad stuff from those sweet treats — like refined flour, sugar, and fat — and just eat the healthy fruits and veggies hiding inside, those delicious garden goodies might keep that middle-age spread at bay.

It's every dieter's dream. Eat as much as you want — without having to count calories. And you can do just that if you fill your plate with nutrient-dense,

How do slim people stay that way? The Global Healthy Weight Registry listed these tips from its members — 96 percent eat breakfast, 69 percent exercise at least three times each week, 65 percent include vegetables with dinner every night, and 74 percent rarely diet. Simple advice. Eat smart, keep moving.

low-calorie fruits and vegetables. When it comes to beating hunger pangs, vegetables and fruits deliver a one-two-three punch.

▶ Plant foods are, on average, 80 to 90 percent water. So when you dig into that plate of fresh veggies, most of what you're eating is zero-calorie water. You get to eat more food — with no weight worries.

▶ Plant protein — like the kind you find in beans, nuts, and leafy greens — helps release hormones that squash your appetite.

▶ And fiber from those foods slows down digestion and controls your blood sugar level so you feel fuller longer. A real weight-control dynamic duo.

So now you know. You can fill up on healthy, good-for-you fruits and vegetables — and just forget tallying the calories. Go ahead. Live the dream, dieters.

Taste the rainbow and find your weight-loss pot of gold.
Red, blue, green, orange, yellow. Your fruits and vegetables have those bright, healthy hues because they contain really good stuff — natural plant chemicals called polyphenols, like anthocyanins and flavonols. Odd words, for sure, but along with gorgeous colors, they deliver a nutritional wallop.

▶ **Anthocyanins.** Want to maintain your weight — or even drop a few pounds? Think red and blue. Strawberries, blueberries, plums, and red and purple grapes are all chock-full of this heart-healthy polyphenol that not only helps control your weight, but can also protect you from the inflammation that contributes to chronic diseases like diabetes.

▸ **Flavonols.** Whittle your middle while you enjoy onions, leeks, broccoli, beans, and apples. Fruits and vegetables like these contain a type of flavonol called quercetin, which is a mighty anti-inflammatory proven to trim extra inches off your waist.

Rethink that drink to whittle your waist. Have stretchy waistbands become a must-have in your wardrobe? Belt getting a bit snug? Here's a tip. That extra belly fat is the first to go when you do one thing — ditch your diet sodas.

It's a fact. A recent study showed that people who use low-calorie sweeteners, like the kind you find in diet sodas, are more likely to weigh more, have a larger waist circumference, and carry more belly fat — and that's the deadly kind. Visceral fat, the type that masses around internal organs deep within your abdominal cavity, is a strong risk factor for serious medical conditions like diabetes, high blood pressure, and even heart disease.

University of Texas researchers followed more than 400 seniors for nine years, and determined the more diet soda you drink, the more your waistline swells. People who drank diet sodas every day added a belt-busting three inches to their middles. That was more than four times the belly bulge experienced by people who avoided sodas. Even the occasional drinker had to let their belts out by a couple of inches.

Why is your favorite diet beverage causing you to pack on pounds? It may be a gut reaction.

Scientists say phony sweeteners aren't digested in your stomach. Instead, these impostors head straight for your intestines, where millions of bacteria — your microbiome — are hard at work digesting nutrients and storing away energy to use later. The sugar fakers — you know them as aspartame, saccharin, and sucralose, among others — change the balance of bacteria there to promote weight gain.

So can those diet drinks. Instead, refresh yourself the natural way with a cool glass of water. Zero calories, great taste — and a trimmer waist.

Warning

This sweet treat turns sour in your stomach

Sweet-seeking dieters were thrilled by the discovery of a sugar alcohol naturally found in fruits, and used in sugar-free treats like chewing gum and candy. To their delight, it did cause the pounds to drop off steadily. But then things got crazy.

Diarrhea, abdominal pain, and dangerous weight loss — just three of the harmful side effects you might experience with the sugar substitute, sorbitol. Here's one woman's story.

A 21-year-old complained to her doctor about terrible gastrointestinal symptoms. And she was worried because her weight had plummeted — leaving her at just 90 pounds. The doctor was baffled until he discovered she chewed approximately 15 sticks of sorbitol-sweetened gum daily. Once the gum was taken away, her digestive system rebounded, and she regained 15 pounds.

If you think you might be sensitive to sorbitol, check labels on cough syrups, diet drinks, and even ice cream. Beware too much of a good thing.

Follow the 80 percent rule to lose weight — and feel great.
You've heard it a thousand times. You need to burn more calories than you take in.

But do you really know how much you eat? Not everybody wants to drag out the calorie-counting book or look up each food online. You could guess, but, let's face it, looks can be deceiving. Did you know one tiny piece of your favorite candy can set you back a good 300 calories?

Wait a minute. Suppose you had an internal calorie-meter that would let you know when you've eaten enough? Well, you do. Just pay attention to your stomach. The long-lived Okinawans have been doing it for generations.

Hara hachi bu. Three magic words that mean eat only until you are 80 percent full. Or, to put it more bluntly, don't stuff yourself. The people of Okinawa recite this mantra before meals as a reminder to practice self-control. Give it a try. You have nothing to lose — but a few more pounds.

The bottom line is to pay attention while you're eating. Tricks like repeating hara hachi bu before a meal can help you cut your calorie intake. Here are some other tips for mindful eating.

▸ When you sit down to eat, think about how your stomach feels. On a scale of one to 10, how hungry are you? Next, stop halfway through your meal and reassess. Are you still hungry, or have you hit your 80-percent mark?

▸ Eat slowly. It takes about 20 minutes for your brain to get the message your hunger is satisfied. Put your fork down between bites. Give your body time to get in sync.

▶ Gauge your fullness factor. Try this. Stand up partway through your meal to see how you feel. Comfortably full? You've eaten enough. Feeling bloated? You've gone overboard. Learn your body's fullness signals.

▶ Focus on your food — not your screens. Turn off the TV and mute your cellphone. Instead, savor each bite and enjoy the experience.

Fast-track your weight loss with exercise. You know why you're overweight — too many calories in, not enough energy out. It's pretty simple. So why can't you lose the extra weight despite your best efforts to eat less?

Blame it on your genes. The FTO gene, located on your 16th chromosome, to be exact. Researchers have discovered that people with this gene have a harder time peeling off the pounds. And the best way to beat it? Exercise. That's right. Scientists found that regular exercise can lessen the effect of FTO by up to 75 percent.

An hour of exercise each week is all it takes. A three-year study of more than 17,000 people showed just one hour a week of aerobic exercise — like jogging or swimming — was more beneficial for weight loss than dieting.

But what if you don't have the knees for jogging or there's no pool nearby? You can get in that 60-minute workout lots of different ways. Go for any exercise that:

▶ involves a steady, rhythmic activity.

▶ includes large muscle groups like your arms and legs.

▶ makes your lungs work hard.

Try some brisk walking, cycling, dancing, or step aerobics. Be sure to pick something you enjoy so you'll stick with it.

The benefits add up, too. Besides trimming off the extra pounds, studies prove with exercise you can beat the symptoms of depression, lower your risk for heart attack and stroke, and drop those blood pressure numbers.

First things first, though. Make sure you check with your doctor before you begin a new exercise program.

Don't fall for this dieting slip-up

Who Knew?

You take a snack with you on your walk to quell those hunger pangs, but that may actually derail your weight loss.

Researchers studied 60 women who were given cereal bars to munch while they took a walk, talked to a friend, or watched TV. Later, they had seven minutes to eat as much of the following foods as they wanted — carrot sticks, M&M's, grapes, or chips.

Bet you think the TV group ate the most, right? Nope. The walking group ate more — including five times more chocolate. Why? Researchers think snacking while walking may not register in your brain as eating, but as exercise, instead. So you feel justified in indulging in a favorite snack.

Paying attention to what and when you eat, experts say, is important for successful weight management.

Lose more weight with a bowl, a spoon, and this superfood. It can melt away belly fat in just five minutes each morning — no sit-ups needed. Plus you can get it at the corner grocery.

What is this amazing solution to staying slim? Whole grains, like the kind you find in ready-to-eat breakfast cereals. That's it. Studies prove that women who eat one, two, and even three servings of high-fiber, whole grains each day are less likely to be overweight than women who eat no whole grains.

With whole-grain foods, you're treated to a taste of all three parts of the grain — the germ, the endosperm, and the bran. None of the good stuff is left out. And these high-fiber foods — like whole-grain breads and cereals — help fill you up and keep you feeling full longer. So you eat less.

But a slimmer waist is not the only benefit. Fill up on healthy whole grains and you might even live longer, since you're getting a heaping helping of protection from heart disease, pneumonia, and other infections. Turns out the fiber in whole grain cereals, for example, helps regulate blood pressure, lower cholesterol, and reduce inflammation that can lead to respiratory diseases.

Trim fat and calories with this easy-as-pie tip. Don't let that piece of pepperoni pizza blow your diet. Just dab it with a napkin to get off the excess grease. Some say you'll cut around 40 calories — and more than 4 grams of fat — per slice. Pizza night is saved.

So which foods give you the most whole grain goodness? They can be a little tricky to spot. Start by reading labels carefully.

The first ingredient should say 100 percent whole wheat, oats, barley, or some other grain. If you see the words "whole grain" on a product, then it must contain a minimum of 51 percent whole grain ingredients by weight per serving.

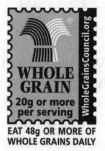

The stamp from the Whole Grains Council is one way to tell if a food does indeed contain whole grains. Look for it before you buy.

A healthier life, 15 minutes at a time. Can you spare 15 minutes out of your busy day to improve your health? Start your stopwatch. These three timely tips will put those precious moments to good use.

> ▶ **Walk it off.** Researchers say a 15-minute walk after each meal, especially dinner, helps regulate your blood sugar — even better than one long 45-minute walk. And it burns up a few calories to boot. If you're a 154-pound man, a brisk after-meal walk will burn about 70 calories. That means in just one year you could feel fitter, livelier — and 7 pounds lighter.

> ▶ **Write it down.** A recent study said people who kept a daily food journal lost twice as much weight as those who didn't. So take 15 minutes each day to write down the foods you've eaten, the portion sizes, the time of day — even your mood. Include BLTs, too. That's bites, licks, and tastes. And don't forget to list beverages. Those liquid calories can add up quickly.

> Write in your journal faithfully, and it will provide an accurate record of what food is going in your mouth, when it's

going in, and why. A great tool to help you create a tasty, healthful meal plan just right for you.

▶ **Talk it over.** Researchers agree that emotional support from friends and family will help you stick to your new lifestyle. One study found that people who enrolled in a weight-management program with friends did a better job of keeping their weight off. In other words, you need a team you can count on.

So maybe you didn't eat very well today. Take 15 minutes to call a friend and talk over your diet distress. Or maybe you crashed on the couch instead of heading out to an aerobics class. Use those 15 minutes to find a weight management group that can get you motivated. Some are free, others charge a nominal membership fee, and some organizations offer a buffet of services and prices. Contact your local hospital or community education center for groups near you.

It's quick and easy to make a change for the better. All you need is 15 minutes.

Rx Alert: just say no to dangerous diet drugs

Nausea. Headache. Suicidal thoughts. Increased risk of heart attack and stroke. Just a few of the many side effects associated with weight loss medications. The following eight drugs have been approved by the FDA for weight management, but that doesn't mean they are right for you.

Generic	Brand name(s)	Possible side effects	How it works
benz-phetamine	Didrex	hallucinations, nervousness, high blood pressure, severe headache, slurred speech, blurred vision, and seizure	This drug may decrease your appetite, increase the amount of energy used by your body, or affect certain parts of your brain to control hunger.
diethyl-propion	Tenuate	anxiety, dizziness, hair loss, chest pain, shortness of breath, and seizures	It works by suppressing the appetite center in your brain to temporarily reduce hunger.
lorcaserin	Belviq	dizziness, fatigue, memory problems, and heart valve trouble	It works by increasing feelings of fullness so you eat less food.
naltrexone and bu-propion	Contrave	suicidal thoughts, increased blood pressure, and risk of seizures	Bupropion is an antide-pressant that can also decrease appetite. Naltrexone may curb hunger and food cravings.
orlistat	Xenical, Alli	gas, leaky bowel movements, and liver damage	It slows the absorption of fat in your intestine.
phendi-metrazine	Plegine, Bontril PDM	fainting, chest pain, irregular heartbeat, headache, and fatal lung or heart problems	Phendimetrazine increases your heart rate and blood pressure, and decreases your appetite.
phentermine	Adipex, Fastin	high blood pressure, dizziness, chest pain, and addiction	Phentermine is supposed to increase your feelings of fullness and reduce cravings.
phentermine and topira-mate	Qysmia	increased heart rate, depression, anxiety, and insomnia	These medicines work in your brain to make you less interested in food.

Fish oil lights your fat-burning fire

Who Knew?

You take fish oil to fight heart disease and lower cholesterol, but who knew it could turn your fat-storing cells into fat-burning cells?

Your body has three kinds of fat cells.

- White fat is the kind you want to get rid of because it basically just sits there and stores fat.

- Brown fat burns energy to regulate body temperature. Babies have lots of brown fat, but it typically goes away as you age.

- Beige fat can essentially change from white to brown during times of stress, like when you are cold.

When it's time to burn fat, your body releases a special protein that fires up the brown cells. Researchers discovered when fish oil was added to the diet, this protein also appeared in white cells. Their theory? Fish oil can transform your fat-storage cells into fat-scorcher cells. Holy mackerel.

Power through the weight-loss plateau

You step up on the scale. You suck in your breath — along with your stomach — and peer down at your feet. Gasp. You haven't dropped an ounce. In weeks. Oh, no. Looks like you've hit the dreaded diet plateau.

Here's why your weight loss has come to a screeching halt. It's all about metabolism, or the number of calories you burn on a daily basis. See, the more body mass you have, the more calories you burn. That's why it was easy to lose weight those first few weeks. But now that some pounds have dropped off, your metabolism has slowed down. And that means slower weight loss.

A weight-loss plateau like this occurs when the number of calories you eat is the same as the number you burn. Now that you aren't burning calories as quickly or easily, you have to amp it up.

Try these quick ways to unstick your scale and turn your body back into that lean, mean, fat-fighting machine.

▸ **Check your records.** Are you keeping a food journal? Look it over to make sure you haven't increased your portion sizes or snuck some unhealthy snacks into your diet.

▸ **Cut a few more calories.** Sure it's tough, but even 200 fewer every day can make a difference. Don't go below a daily total of 1,200 calories, though. If you don't eat enough, you'll feel hungry all the time — increasing the likelihood you'll make bad food choices.

▸ **Punch up your daily activity by 15 to 30 minutes.** And don't forget to add a little strength training. It helps build muscle, and muscle tissue burns more calories than fat.

Now read about three amazing beverages that will help you push past your weight-loss plateau.

Slim down with water. Here's a weight-loss stunner. Researchers found that drinking just 4 ounces of H2O, 20 minutes before meals, stimulates weight loss — even if you do nothing else. And a study of more than 18,000 adults showed that people who drank one to three cups of plain, ordinary water daily knocked up to 200 calories off their total intake.

Experts think some of the extra calories burn up as your body heats the water. But all that water makes you feel fuller, too, and that helps you eat less.

Cure deadly belly fat with vinegar. Good old-fashioned vinegar — a diluted form of acetic acid — signals your body to flip the switch from storing fat to burning fat.

A recent Japanese study found that taking two tablespoons of apple cider vinegar every day for 12 weeks — mixed in a specially prepared beverage — helped people lose five pounds and trim nearly an inch from around their middles. Best of all, without doing anything else different, they lost dangerous visceral fat that builds up around your internal organs.

Experts think vinegar slows down food as it travels through your stomach — so you can go longer without feeling hungry. And apple cider vinegar may contain a small amount of a fiber called pectin that's known to help you feel full longer.

But remember, never drink vinegar straight since it can irritate your throat and mouth. And because it can interact with medications like diuretics and insulin, talk to your doctor before you add it to your daily routine.

Conquer your plateau with a cup of tea. Nudge the scale with one of the oldest and most popular beverages in the world. Researchers found that drinking four cups of green tea every day led to significant weight loss — and a slimmer waist — among adults with type 2 diabetes.

Experts believe it's the natural plant chemicals, polyphenols like epigallocatechin gallate (EGCG), that may keep your body from digesting and absorbing starch — a type of carbohydrate known to pack on the pounds.

An added bonus? Green tea's powerful antioxidants can also drop your blood pressure and even help control your cholesterol.

Just don't go overboard. Studies show three to five cups of green tea a day is considered safe, but you can damage your liver with high doses of green tea extract supplements.

Is your bacteria making you fat?

Quick! Name three things that are contagious. Yawning. Laughter. The common cold. All good answers. But what about obesity? Bet you didn't think of that one. Yet today's scientists are speculating you can "catch" obesity from your family members.

So does that mean you can blame your extra pounds on Mom's genes? Not exactly. Your weight troubles might actually have less to do with her genes — and more to do with her gut.

Your microbial makeup — a world within. Your bowel is a happening place. It's part of your microbiome, a mini-ecosystem packed full of bacteria ready to help digest food, destroy organisms that cause disease, metabolize drugs, prevent infection, and provide you with nutrients.

You picked up some of your mother's intestinal bacteria as you passed through the birth canal. In fact, that's how you began your own personal gut flora. But since then, you've added many more bacteria — trillions of them — making your microbiome as unique as your fingerprint. So what does this have to do with weight?

The great bacteria battle rages on. Right now bacteria are fighting it out in your digestive tract, with two types, Bacteroidetes and Firmicutes, as the major opposing armies.

▶ Bacteroidetes, the good guys, are fiber-eating bacteria that work to keep you slim and trim. They specialize in breaking down bulky plant starches and fibers into shorter molecules your body uses for energy.

▶ Firmicutes — remember F for "fat" — can actually hijack your appetite and turn you into a bulging fat-storage machine. They take the rubbish from the foods you eat, break it down, and release those calories back into your bloodstream. In other words, calories that should end up as waste, instead end up on your waist — and your thighs, and your hips. You get the picture. All because of Firmicutes.

Scientists have figured out that people who have more Firmicutes than Bacteroidetes in their microbiome are more likely to be obese.

So are the extra pounds around your middle caused by your mother's — or father's — Firmicutes? Could be. Studies show that you share many of your microbes with your entire household — even the family dog. Don't point that finger of blame just yet, though. More research needs to be done before scientists know for sure.

Antibiotics — when the war on bugs goes awry. Remember, the purpose of antibiotics is to kill bacteria. And they are quite good at their job. Maybe too good. More often than not, they blast the beneficial bacteria right along with the bad. When the bacteria balance in your microbiome is changed in this way, the out-of-whack gut germs not only affect the Bacteroidetes Firmicutes ratio, but can set you up for serious health problems like colon cancer, diabetes, Crohn's disease, and ulcerative colitis.

Certain kinds of bad bacteria can also promote the inflammation that contributes to diseases affecting your skin, lungs, and joints — like rheumatoid arthritis. Researchers have even found links between the metabolites produced in your microbiome to brain issues — think anxiety, depression, autism, and Alzheimer's disease.

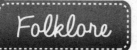

Why 3,500 calories doesn't always equal 1 pound

It's a dieter's rule of thumb. Cut 3,500 calories out of your weekly diet — that's 500 per day — and you'll lose a pound. But that's not necessarily true, say the experts.

The 3,500-calorie rule doesn't account for important factors like your gender, age, activity level, and amount of fat on your body. Plus, as you trim down, you don't need as many calories to function. You may experience those exciting pound-a-week results at first, but then get discouraged as weight loss slows. Don't give up. There's hope.

Nutritionists and mathematicians put their heads together to develop a personalized calculator to help you achieve your healthy weight. Plug in your numbers, and it will figure out how much exercise you should add every day and how many calories you can subtract. Check it out online at *supertracker.usda.gov/bwp*.

How to build a healthy gut. You truly are what you eat, at least when it comes to your microbiome. So if you're looking for a way to get a better balance of good bacteria in your gut, start first with your diet.

Three delicious foods, in particular, can speed you on your way to good gut health — grapes, apples, and red wine vinegar. All three contain healthy polyphenols, natural plant chemicals that fight off the fat-storing Firmicutes, and feed the keep-you-lean Bacteroidetes.

Here are some other ways you can get your gut back in balance.

▶ **Fill up on fiber.** Women ages 19 to 50 need 25 grams of fiber a day, men 38 grams. However, most get only half that amount. And that's bad news for your microbiome, since fiber is its main source of nutrition.

▶ **Pack in the probiotics.** You can regain control of your gut by adding back the good guys. Probiotic supplements and foods with natural or added probiotics, like cultured dairy drinks, contain live bacteria similar to the good ones that inhabit your gut. Including them in your diet every day floods your intestines with beneficial bacteria that remain active in your digestive tract. Enjoy more fermented foods like yogurt with live and active cultures, homemade sauerkraut, and even some pickles. Talk to your doctor about pairing any antibiotic she prescribes with an over-the-counter probiotic.

▶ **Get plenty of sleep.** Any upset in your sleep cycle can also upset your gut.

▶ **Exercise.** Variety is the key to good gut health. When it comes to belly bacteria, the more kinds you have the better. If your bowel has a large variety of bacteria, it can break down lots of different foods into small molecules — called metabolites — that help both your immune system and your brain function properly. One study found athletes had more diversity in their microbiomes than their less-athletic buddies. For better belly bacteria, schedule a good-for-your-gut walk around the block every day.

This time, keep the weight off — for good

Popular humorist Erma Bombeck lamented, "In two decades I've lost a total of 789 pounds. I should be hanging from a charm bracelet." Can you relate? If you're like most dieters, you know exactly what she means. You repeatedly lose and regain those same, infuriating pounds. What's going on?

Medical professionals call it weight cycling. You may know it as yo-yo dieting. And it's caused by a drop in your resting metabolic rate (RMR) — the number of calories your body burns just for basic processes, like breathing and circulation.

The more weight you lose, the fewer calories your body needs to maintain the slimmer, trimmer you, and the lower your RMR. But unless you adjust your calories, your weight sneaks back up. You can't eat like you did before you lost weight. And that's where most folks run into trouble.

But you can cut that yo-yo string forever with these tips.

Don't ever diet again. Instead, create a meal plan that you can stick to — and enjoy — for life. Try experimenting with new, good-for-you recipes. But choose lots of different kinds of foods to add to your menus. In one study, people who increased the variety of healthy foods in their meal plan lost the most weight and were the most successful in maintaining their new weight two years later.

Make sure your plan includes fruits and vegetables with lots of flavonoids like apigenin, found in parsley and celery, and naringenin, plentiful in grapefruit juice. Research shows these two flavonoids keep your gut's microbiome healthy and your weight steady.

Avoid rebound pounds with exercise. Researchers at the University of Alabama found women who lost weight then participated in exercise — especially weight training — burned more calories during the day, which helped them keep their weight off.

And members of The National Weight Control Registry — more than 10,000 people who have lost at least 30 pounds and kept it off for a year or more — recommend you exercise one hour a day to maintain your weight. Their favorite activity? Nothing fancy. Just brisk walking.

Keep bad eating habits at bay. Continue to write in your food journal, and beware of those trigger foods that tempt you to overeat. Weigh yourself on a regular basis, and spring into action if the scale goes up more than five pounds. Finally, surround yourself with friends and family who will help you maintain your weight — and support your new, healthy lifestyle.

C